TOTAL HEART RATE
TRAINING

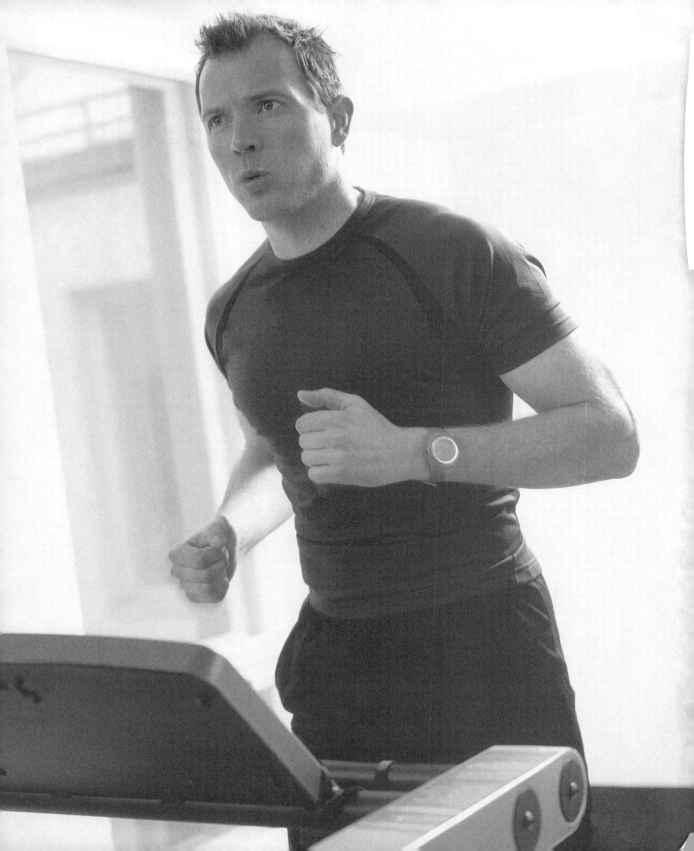

TOTAL HEART RATE TRAINING

Customize and Maximize Your Workout Using a Heart Rate Monitor

JOE FRIEL

Ulysses Press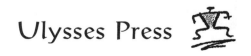

Published in the U.S. by Ulysses Press
P.O. Box 3440
Berkeley, CA 94703
www.ulyssespress.com

ISBN10: 1-56975-562-0
ISBN13: 978-1-56975-562-4
Library of Congress Control Number 2006903820

Printed in Canada by Webcom

10 9 8 7 6 5 4 3 2

Managing Editor: Claire Chun
Editor: Lily Chou
Copyeditor: Mark Woodworth
Editorial Associates: Rebekah Morris, Elyce Petker, Stefanie Tamura
Index: Sayre Van Young
Production: Matt Orendorff, Steven Zah Schwartz
Cover design: what!design @ whatweb.com
Cover photos: cyclist and woman on treadmill © iStockphoto.com; runner © Polar
Interior design: Lourdes Robles
Indexer: Sayre Van Young
Photographs: © Polar

Distributed by Publishers Group West

Please Note
This book has been written and published strictly for informational purposes, and in no way should be used as a substitute for consultation with health care professionals. You should not consider educational material herein to be the practice of medicine or to replace consultation with a physician or other medical practitioner. The author and publisher are providing you with information in this work so that you can have the knowledge and can choose, at your own risk, to act on that knowledge. The author and publisher also urge all readers to be aware of their health status and to consult health care professionals before beginning any health program.

TABLE OF CONTENTS

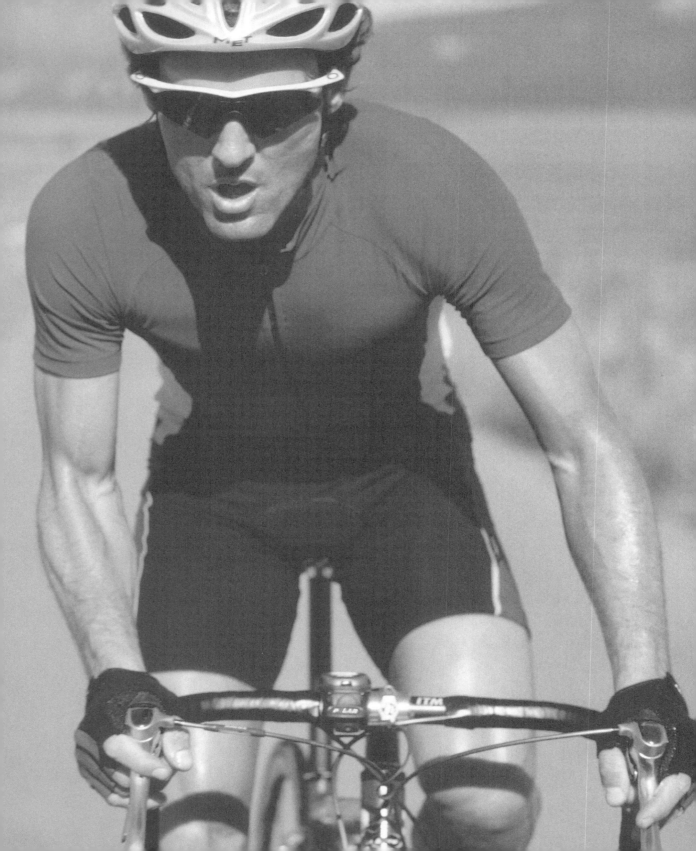

PREFACE

That you are reading this book says a lot about you. You are an athlete with a desire to perform at a higher level. You undoubtedly already own a heart rate monitor and may have been using it for some time—perhaps even years. You strap it on every day as you head out the door for your workout. You've been using it for so long that it would feel strange not to have it on. But you still sense a bit of mystery surrounding its use. So your desire to race faster and your inquisitiveness have led you to this book.

Purchasing and reading a book is a commitment of both money and time on your part that I take very seriously. I want this book to be worth your investment. You should come away from it with answers to many heart rate training questions, including some you may not even be aware of yet. You probably have some basic questions right now about this book. Let's answer them.

First of all, why is this book called *TOTAL Heart Rate Training*? Why not just call it *Heart Rate Training*? The reason is that I wrote this book to venture well beyond what other authors have already said so well when describing the basics of training by heart rate. *Total Heart Rate Training* will teach you how to integrate heart rate and other methods of measuring intensity into a periodized training plan based on your unique needs. It contains a thorough and complete description of the training process, written from a heart rate perspective.

Can this book help you? Will you be faster? Will you endure long races, better than ever? The answer, as with all such questions, begins with "it depends…." For starters, it depends on how dedicated you are to closely following the program that will be laid out for you in Chapter 9. It depends on whether you will even take the time to create such a personalized program. Can this book help you? I have no doubt that it can.

I've been coaching endurance athletes for a wide variety of sports since 1980, using the principles described on the following pages. I've worked with hundreds of athletes, both men and women, with a wide range of ages and abilities. Their sports have been running, swimming, road cycling, mountain biking, triathlon, duathlon, rowing, and endurance horse racing. The *Total Heart Rate Training* program has worked for all of them.

The athletes I've coached using what is described here have included a World Champion, an Olympian, several world-class performers, national champions, top regional competitors, age-group winners, first-time finishers, and those who have dramatically improved their performances. These people were all dedicated to the program.

Don't get me wrong, there have been a few who did not improve, who believed they could modify the program and perform better that way. These athletes seldom performed to expectations. But those who followed the program performed remarkably well. You cannot make sweeping changes to this program and expect it to work better for you. It has too many interconnected parts. It would be like trying to change the inner workings of a watch to make it run better. You might get away with it for a while, but eventually the changes will catch up with you and performance will decline.

Can using a heart rate monitor help you perform better? *Anyone* participating in aerobic sports, from novice to expert, can benefit from paying attention to heart rate during exercise. Heart rate serves as a window into the body, telling you what your physical and mental systems are experiencing based on all the factors affecting them—exercise intensity, diet, temperature and humidity, altitude, fatigue, and more. Wearing a heart rate monitor is like having a coach along for the workout, who tells you when to go harder and when to back off. Computer software makes training analysis a snap. And with the advent of other intensity-measuring devices in the last few years, heart rate monitoring is even more effective now than it ever has been for the seasoned veteran. New gizmos such as powermeters and accelerometers enable you to compare your body's input, as measured by heart rate, with its output—power or pace. The combination makes for precise training that practically guarantees you'll achieve your fitness goals. This book examines all these issues, and more, to guide novices in learning to use a heart rate monitor for the first time, while helping experienced athletes get more benefit from the heart rate monitors they have been using for a long time.

I've had a lot of experience using a heart rate monitor, both as an athlete and as a coach. It was 1983 when I first saw a wireless heart rate monitor. At the time I owned the first triathlon store in the United States, perhaps in the world. (It was way too early for that sport to support such a business, but that's another story.) We sold swim, bike, and run gear not only to triathletes but also to swimmers, cyclists, and runners. The store's employees were all serious athletes, and some were also grad students at Colorado State University in Fort Collins. The store, called Foot of the Rockies, was right next to the campus.

We were always on the lookout for anything that could help make us better athletes, and we frequently argued the relative merits of training in particular ways. Heart rate was an underlying theme of many of our discussions. It seemed to be such an obvious thing—count your pulse, and use that as a precise and perhaps perfect way of judging how hard we were training. Getting an accurate number, though, was always the problem. By the time we stopped swimming, biking, or running and found our pulse at the throat, it had already begun to drop. While we counted, it dropped even lower. It just wasn't very precise.

Then one day a sales representative came into the store with a heart rate monitor. It was a Polar Sport Tester PE-2000. I still have it. By today's standards it was a clunker, but at the time it seemed like a technological marvel. Here was a device you could wear during a workout or race and it would display your heart rate *while you were exercising!* It was space-age stuff.

I bought several for the store and one for myself. At first I had no idea what the numbers meant. Was 160 good or bad? Why was heart rate on the bike lower than when running, even though both seemed hard? I had a lot more questions than answers. I recall wearing it all day just to watch my heart rate, and liked to show it off to other athletes. I'd brush my teeth with it on to see what happened. As I walked up stairs I'd look to see how fast heart rate rose and how quickly it came down when I reached the top. While watching TV I'd reach over and touch my wife to see what my heart did (she didn't like that, but my heart obviously did!).

There were many lessons, and the learning curve was steep for a long time. It took years to figure it out, but by 1987 I had a pretty good idea of what heart rate was telling me. It would be several more years before I knew what it meant relative to pace and power. These lessons, however, were the most important. All the lessons I learned are explained on the following pages.

Heart rate monitors didn't really catch on in the United States for several years. At first there were only a few users, and we were always comparing notes. Occasionally a magazine would run an article on heart rate and we'd read, discuss, and debate the merits of what the author had to say. Then in 1991 a curious thing began to happen. When I went to races—especially triathlon, cycling, and running—I noticed that most of the athletes were wearing heart rate monitors. This was the critical year—some 25 years after they were invented. The tipping point had finally been reached. Not long after that it seemed that everyone was wearing a heart rate monitor. Now they are as ubiquitous as sunglasses at races.

Total Heart Rate Training takes you step by step through the lessons that I learned over 20 years. By the time you have read this book you should have an excellent idea not only of how to train with heart rate, but also simply how to

train. Training today is vastly more complex than it was in 1983. The digital technology explosion has made it possible to train more precisely and effectively—*if* you know how to use the technology.

Heart rate monitors almost seem passé today since they've been around for so long and so many other intensity-measuring devices are available. The interesting thing, though, is that as the number of devices increases, heart rate becomes even more effective. In the old days we had nothing to compare heart rate with to know what it meant. Today you can compare your instantaneous heart rate with your instantaneous pace or power. That exponentially increases the value of your heart rate monitor.

Today if you are a cyclist and don't have a powermeter, or a runner without an accelerometer to go along with your heart rate monitor, then you don't know what you are missing. It reminds me of when I was in high school and thought the world looked a bit fuzzy to everyone, as it did to me. Later, when I got my first pair of glasses, I was amazed to find that the world was actually quite clear. *Why didn't someone tell me?* If you don't have the capability to compare exercise input (heart rate) with output (power or pace), then you simply don't know what you can't see. You'll be as amazed as I was about how the world looks when you correct this discrepancy. "*So that's what training is all about!*" I can imagine you saying.

The first two chapters introduce you to the heart rate monitor and to your heart. Here you'll learn what makes both of them tick. Chapter 3 gets you started using your heart rate monitor, based on the unique system I developed 20 years ago. It's only been slightly modified since then and has pretty much stood the test of time. Chapter 4 takes you beyond the basic lessons taught in the previous chapter. Here you'll learn how to do the power and pace comparisons mentioned earlier, along with many other important lessons. Chapters 5, 6, 7, and 8 take you down the path of how to use your heart rate monitor in various aspects of training. Chapter 9 brings everything together. Here you will complete a workbook type of activity to develop a thorough training plan based on your unique circumstances.

I think you'll find that this book helps you become a fitter and faster athlete. It won't be easy, and you are bound to have questions as you read or begin to apply the principles explained here. If you do, feel free to contact me through my website at www.TotalHRT.com. Let's get started.

Joe Friel
October 2006
Scottsdale, Arizona

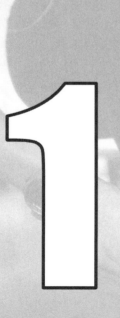

1

YOUR
HEART
RATE
MONITOR

Today we take the heart rate monitor for granted. In fact, monitors are so common now that few athletes today even remember a time when they weren't used. But the older athletes do, and can tell stories of what training was like in those "olden days" before digital technology first appeared, miniaturized, on their wrists. They can also tell you how much fun training became when they got their first heart rate monitors. They talk about wearing it all day at first to see how their daily activities affected heart rate. What numbers would they see when taking the stairs instead of the elevator? How low would their heart rate go while watching an exciting TV show or an action movie? Did brushing their teeth cause heart rate to rise? How about touching their spouse, driving the car, eating, or talking with the boss at work?

You yourself may have tried some of these little tests. If you have, what you discovered is that the heart rate monitor is indeed a wondrous biofeedback tool. If you paid close attention to the numbers and compared them with the activities that produced those numbers, you soon learned how your body responds to all sorts of stresses, both big and little. Even if you have no experience using a monitor, you probably know that exercise is stress. If it weren't, you would have no reason to exercise, and your body wouldn't change by any intentional act. But stress is only half of what ultimately increases your fitness, and it must be great enough to cause the body to adapt. The other half of what increases your fitness is rest. It's during rest periods of low-intensity exercise that those changes that we call "fitness" actually occur in the body. Your heart rate monitor will provide the biofeedback for both high- and low-intensity exercise necessary to make you more fit. It is indeed a powerful training tool, and this book will tell you all about it.

In this chapter we'll examine how your heart rate monitoring tool came to be, how it works, and its many features that are available today. The heart rate monitor has come a long way. It all started in a time long ago when men wore their hair long, women sported miniskirts, society was in upheaval about war and race matters, disco music was king, and Americans walked on the moon—that distant era we call the early 1970s.

THE HISTORY OF THE HEART RATE MONITOR

Heart rate monitoring has a rich history in endurance sports. Long before there were electronic devices, endurance athletes realized that the pulse of their beating heart was closely linked to their exertion and therefore their performance. It was obvious. When they exercised at a high intensity, they felt the rapid pounding of their heart. When they took it easy, their heart beat much more slowly. Endurance athletes would commonly check their pulses at the throat or wrist during exercise, but the problem was that this could only be done by slowing down considerably or by completely stopping. Of course, when exercise intensity decreases, the heart beats more slowly and the pulse also decreases, so the longer one stands with his or her fingers on the neck or wrist the more the pulse rate drops. Counting for a minute was entirely useless. Therefore, to get a fairly accurate number, an athlete had to count for only a few seconds, usually 10, so that pulse couldn't slow too much. Then multiplying by 6 would give an estimate of heart rate—a very rough estimate. Unfortunately, research showed that doing it this way was likely to result in an error of at least 9 beats per minute. Another study showed an error of some 17 beats per minute when manually counting. But what else could an athlete do?

[Treffene's Pulse Meter]

It was obvious to coaches and athletes alike that counting pulse was quite inaccurate and that the medical equipment designed to measure heart rate was too expensive and bulky to lug around. Some sort of small, inexpensive device was needed to check pulse during activity rather than when at rest.

Then in the 1970s two breakthroughs occurred. Early in the decade an Australian exercise physiologist and, later on, internationally renowned swim coach, Robert Treffene, Ph.D., began playing around with pulse rate measurement. He soon came up with a handheld monitor, with electrodes and wires, that a coach on a pool deck could use to check the heart rates of swimmers immediately at the end of an interval as they stopped at the pool wall.

[Seppo's Heart Rate Monitor]

The second breakthrough came in 1977. Professor Seppo Säynäjäkangas (pronounced *say-nay-ya-KONG-us*), a 33-year-old electronics professor at Oulu University in Oulu on the west coast of Finland, was an avid cross-country skier, as many Finns are. In 1976 he wanted to help a local ski coach who was frustrated in his attempts to monitor the heart rates of his aspiring athletes. What the professor came up with was a battery-operated, fingertip pulse meter. He knew he was onto something when the Finnish National Cross Country team wanted to use his device, so in 1977 he formed a company called Polar Electro Oy. Polar introduced its first retail monitor, the Tunturi Pulser, the following year. This was a heart rate monitor with a cable-connected chest belt. Five years later, in 1983, Polar introduced the first wireless heart rate monitor using electric field data transfer— the Sport Tester PE 2000. The next year, the company came out with a device containing a computer interface—the Sport Tester PE 3000. High-tech training had finally arrived.

[Conconi's Test]

Surprisingly, athletes and coaches were slow to adopt the heart rate monitor when it first hit the market. But in 1984 something happened that got a lot of ink in magazines covering all endurance sports. In that year Francesco Moser,

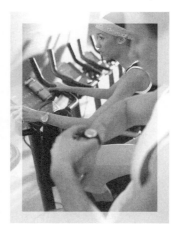

an Italian cyclist, broke Belgian Eddy Merckx's hour record—the distance one could cover in one hour on a track riding solo. Merckx's awesome record distance of 49.431 km (30.746 miles) had been set in 1972 and was thought unbreakable. After all, he was considered the greatest cyclist of all time. Many other excellent cyclists had tried to beat his record, and failed. Moser was considered a decent rider, but not on par with the sport's greats; at the time, he was also approaching the end of his career. But in Mexico City on a cool day in January 1984, in one hour Moser rode 51.151 km (31.815 miles)—a whopping 3 percent farther.

What was interesting about Moser's record attempt was how he trained for it. Until that time riders' training had always been based strictly on perceived exertion—how they felt. Most training was done in groups so that individual riders could push each other to better fitness. Instead of following tradition in his hour-record preparation, Moser trained under the tutelage of an Italian physician—Francesco Conconi.

Dr. Conconi was an early adopter of Säynäjäkangas' heart rate monitor and, in using it for his own running, had made an interesting discovery. When graphing his running paces and heart rates after a track workout in which pace increased gradually every lap, he saw what he believed to be an intriguing phenomenon. When he connected the dots of his graphed pace–heart rate data, the resulting line rose fairly straight from the lower left corner to the upper right. That part was expected. But as the line approached the top end it did something interesting—it bent downward slightly like a stick that had been broken. Conconi believed the point of deflection was the "anaerobic threshold" (later research would cast doubt on this "discovery"). The "Conconi Test" was born.

Conconi knew that a human could maintain anaerobic threshold (AT) effort for about an hour. So when Moser came to him seeking guidance to train for the hour record, the doctor already knew how to prepare for it—use a heart rate monitor, conduct a Conconi Test to pinpoint AT, and then train a lot at that specific heart rate. It worked.

Reading all the hoopla in the press about Moser and Conconi, cyclists, runners, swimmers, cross-country skiers, and other endurance athletes all around the world decided to try heart rate training. The Conconi Test was described and lauded in magazines in many languages and time zones. A new way of training had been born.

HOW THEY WORK

A heart rate monitor has two basic components—a transmitter strapped to the chest and a wristwatch receiver. The chest strap is the more critical piece, as it detects the heart's electrical activity and wirelessly transmits it to the receiver. Several research studies have shown there is no significant difference between heart rates detected and transmitted by telemetric heart rate monitors that a runner in her nylon shorts can wear and an expensive lab setup of hardwired electrocardiograph (ECG) equipment. These studies have found there is about a plus or minus 1 percent difference in accuracy during steady state activity—an insignificant rate. Heart rate monitors are so advanced these days that they are often used in the medical field, primarily because of their accuracy, ease of use, and cost relative to expensive dedicated medical equipment.

Another type of heart rate monitor, marketed to athletes, uses photo-optic sensors, also called infrared, to sense blood flow to a fingertip or earlobe. Familiar to anyone who has been treated in a hospital lately, these are actually "pulse meters," not heart rate monitors, as they measure pulse, not heart rate. When used by athletes outdoors they are not very accurate, owing to changes in light that can interrupt their sensing capability. Movement can also cause interference. While generally less expensive, infrared pulse meters are just not as effective for athletic use. The slightly greater cost of the heart rate monitor is worth it, since reliability and accuracy are critical to serious training.

[The Transmitter]

The chest strap transmitter is the workhorse of a heart rate monitor. It contains two electrodes that sense the electrical activity of the heart through the skin. A small radio transmitter, built into the chest strap, sends the data to the receiver on your wrist or handlebars for display,

data storage, and in-workout analysis. In the "olden days" (ca. 1980s), all chest strap transmitters worked with all receivers. The result was overlapping-display problems when two or more athletes were near each other. Very high and erratic numbers were displayed in such a situation. By the 1990s, some transmitters had been designed to send coded data that could only be "seen" by a similarly coded receiver. Today some receivers work by detecting and displaying either coded or uncoded transmissions, although coded data is preferable.

Even with coding it is still possible to get erroneous data displayed on your receiver. Common culprits are computers, cell phones, high-voltage power lines, cars, and motor-driven exercise equipment. Oddly enough, a light nylon jacket or jersey flapping in a strong wind will mess up the signal, somehow deflecting it. You can also get a jumbled heart rate display, especially early in the workout, if the chest strap is not wet enough. This is most likely to happen on a cold day when you are not sweating and the strap wasn't prepared with enough moisture before putting it on.

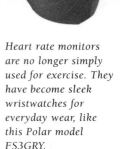

Heart rate monitors are no longer simply used for exercise. They have become sleek wristwatches for everyday wear, like this Polar model FS3GRY.

[The Receiver]

The wristwatch receiver has come a long way since I got my first one back in 1983. In those days receivers were big and cumbersome. You'd never wear it as an everyday watch. They were simply ugly, like early-model remote controls and mobile phones. Today, though, you'll see (or, more likely, *won't* see) athletes wearing their heart rate monitors at the farmer's market and even at formal affairs. They are sleek and elegant. In fact, you can often spot other athletes by the high-tech wristwatches they choose to wear.

HEART RATE MONITOR FEATURES

The functional features of heart rate monitors have also come a long way since the 1970s. Originally, monitors showed only one's instantaneous heart rate—how fast the heart is beating right now. But today's model offers many features, including the following, depending on which monitor you choose.

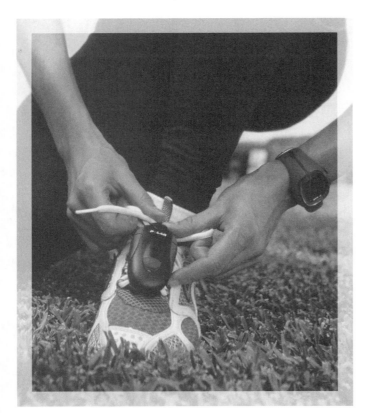

The foot pod accurately measures pace for running and walking.

HEART RATE This is the most basic feature and is found on all devices.

TIME OF DAY Besides time of day, many also feature dual time zones for convenience when traveling.

MEMORY As you work out with your heart rate monitor, it stores time as being in, below, or above your heart rate zone (or zones). Many receivers can store the data relative to three zones that you preset. Later I'll show you how to set this feature relative to your own zones.

STOPWATCH The stopwatch mode is used to time your workout and can also record lap or "split" times for later review. This is useful when you're doing interval workouts and want to record important points, such as mileage markers, during races.

ALARMS Not only do most monitors provide an alarm clock to make sure you wake up in time for your workout, they also offer target zone alarms. These notify you when you are out of the targeted training or racing zone. In effect, they're like a green flag saying, "Hurry up!"

TIMERS Some units have independent countdown or count-up timers. This can be especially helpful during long races to remind you to eat or drink.

CALORIES BURNED You often want to keep track of how many calories you burn while training, so as to keep your body weight in check by balancing output with input. Caloric cost is also a way of gauging the total stress of a workout relative to other workouts. A total of all calories expended for a week can also offer a comparison of how well you are balancing stress with rest. Chapter 7 discusses this.

FITNESS MEASUREMENT Chapter 4 describes field tests you can do to gauge changes in your performance. Polar has also come up with an easy way to measure basic cardiovascular fitness. The Polar "Fitness Test," which some of the manufacturer's units offer as a feature, is done while lying down and is based on your gender, age, height, and body weight, plus your level of physical activity, your heart rate, and your heart rate variability. The result is displayed as your "OwnIndex"—a number between 20 and 95. The company offers a standard scale for comparison. For example, a score of 20 indicates an unfit, sedentary individual while a 95 represents the fitness level of an Olympic athlete.

PACE For a runner or walker, the most valuable data besides heart rate is pace or power—how fast they are moving. Global Positioning Satellite (GPS) systems have been available for outdoor athletes for several years. The problem with them, however, is that when you are in a place where you don't have line-of-sight positioning with a satellite, as when in a forest or a city with tall buildings, they simply don't work. A more recent innovation that resolves this dilemma is the accelerometer. Polar's accelerometer uses a "foot pod" that clips onto your running shoe's laces and transmits speed and distance data to the wristwatch receiver, where it is displayed along with heart rate. After calibration it measures foot acceleration and deceleration to calculate your velocity and distance with 99 percent accuracy.

BICYCLE SPEED AND DISTANCE Heart rate is also found on some bicycle handlebar computers, along with standard data such as speed, distance, and time. This data is usually calculated by way of a small magnet mounted on the spokes of the front wheel. The data is detected by a sensor and transmitted to the handlebars, where it is shown on a small computer screen.

BICYCLE POWER When riding a bike out on the road or up a trail, speed means little to you since it is greatly affected by wind and terrain. While heart rate tells you what your "input" is, it doesn't tell you anything about "output"—how much work you are producing. That's where power comes in. Power for cycling is roughly the equivalent of pace for running. It is not affected by wind or terrain. The problem with most powermeters is their cost— expect to pay more than $1,000. Polar has brought the price way down with their "Power Output Sensor" technology, an ingenious device that measures the vibrations of the chain as it passes through a sensor fastened on the bicycle's right-side chain stay and sends the information to a handlebar receiving device (which also doubles as a wristwatch off the bike). Besides power, it displays pedaling cadence, speed, time, and, of course, heart rate as transmitted from a chest strap. This device will cost you a third or less of the price of the most basic, traditional powermeter. It's a great way to get started training with power.

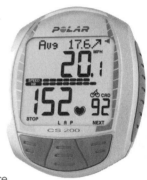

The Polar CS200.

ALTITUDE Now we're getting into features that are found on very few heart rate monitors but may prove useful nevertheless. Take altitude, for example. If you often train or race on hilly terrain, it can prove insightful to know how much climbing and descending you're doing. You certainly know that a workout with a lot of ups and downs is far different from a flat workout. If you spend a lot of time at elevations above about 8,000 feet, as in Colorado's Rocky Mountains, knowing how quickly you are ascending can help you avoid acute mountain sickness. And, besides, simply knowing your altitude at any given time is fun and really impresses your training partners.

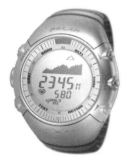

The Polar AXN700 displays not only heart rate but also altitude, barometric pressure, and temperature. It even has a compass.

BAROMETRIC PRESSURE Heart rate monitors that display altitude usually also show barometric pressure, since the latter is often used to determine elevation. This function can even predict and notify you when bad weather is on the way, giving you time to seek shelter.

TEMPERATURE How hot or cold is it during your workout? It's amazing, I know, but some heart rate monitors will even tell you this. For accuracy's sake, though, it's best to take the watch off your wrist before taking a reading, so that body temperature doesn't interfere with the reading.

COMPASS Have you ever gotten lost on a long workout in a strange place? Here's the solution: Get a heart rate monitor that comes equipped with a compass. Columbus was never so lucky.

GRAPHICAL DISPLAYS Receivers are getting so sophisticated these days that the distinction between their in-workout displays and the analysis software with which they come packaged is fading. Many devices now produce a mini-graph, along with various functions. For example, some provide a visual display of how your heart rate varies throughout a workout, or show how altitude or barometric pressure has changed during your session.

COMPUTER UPLOAD Many heart rate monitors are now so high-tech that they can even easily download data to your computer for post-workout analysis. The software will often do the analysis for you (no hands needed). The download is done by a pluggable modem or an infrared interface. If you have a coach, you now have a great way to tell him or her what happened, simply by sending your file after a race or workout. A website that offers a wide range of analysis functionality and is compatible with most heart rate monitors and other devices such as powermeters and handlebar computers is www.trainingbible.com.

Polar also offers a free training diary and other analysis options for its devices at www.polar.fi.

THE **HEART OF THE** MATTER

Athletes have probably been checking their pulses for as long as endurance competition has been going on, because there is an obvious link between exercise intensity and how fast the heart beats. While the electronic heart rate monitor has been around since the early 1970s, it took a decade before models were sufficiently streamlined and functional to be commonly used by endurance athletes. The two components of a heart rate monitor are the chest strap, which senses the electrical activity of the heart and transmits the data to the other component, a wristwatch or handlebar receiver, where it is interpreted and displayed. Heart rate monitors now come with many features beyond simply displaying heart rate and include a wide array of functions such as time of day, memory, stopwatch, alarms, timers, calories burned, fitness measurement, pace, speed and distance, bicycle power, altitude, barometric pressure, temperature, compass, graphic displays, and computer upload capabilities.

YOUR **2** HEART RATE

There is no doubt that the invention of the wireless heart rate monitor has changed the way that endurance athletes both train and race. The average athlete today is much more knowledgeable about what's going on in their body than the sharpest athletes were 30 years ago. There is still considerable room for improvement, however. In this chapter I want to introduce you to your heart and, more specifically, to your heart rate.

I hear many comments and complaints about heart rate from athletes. Here are some of the common ones, along with what the athlete really means. Each is based on a faulty understanding of the exercising heart rate. By the end of this chapter you should be able to detect the underlying error of each.

- "My heart rate is too high!" (Translation: There's something wrong with me!)

- "My heart rate won't go up!" (Translation: I'm in bad shape!)

- "I hit my zones easily!" (Translation: I'm in great shape!)

- "My heart rate is lower than yours!" (Translation: I'm a loser!)

- "My zones are easier when I run than when I swim!" (Translation: Isn't that great!)

THE CARDIOVASCULAR SYSTEM

The heart is a marvelous device. It works non-stop (we hope!) day after day for years. Its endurance capability is amazing. Try using any other muscle in your body in this same way and see what happens.

Like other muscles in the body the heart grows larger and stronger when stressed. When not stressed, as when its owner sits in front of the TV day after day, it shrivels up just as other muscles do. The heart can use carbohydrate, fat, or lactate for fuel equally well. To produce energy, the heart muscles are literally packed with little energy-producing organs called "mitochondria." About 25 to 30 percent of the couch potato's heart muscle cells are made up of these tiny powerhouses. For comparison, the biceps muscle of an untrained person is about 5 percent mitochondria.

An athlete's heart does not have the ability to beat any faster than a spectator's. Ounce for ounce, the world-class athlete's heart doesn't create any more muscular force than anyone else's heart. The number of mitochondria is not any greater in the heart muscle of the winner of the race than those in the heart muscle of the last-place finisher.

[The Pump]

The heart is first and foremost a pump, and as with any pump there are only two ways to increase its output. One is to keep the chamber the same size but to pump faster. The other is to keep the stroke rate the same, but to increase the size of the chamber so that more fluid is pumped per stroke. The latter is more efficient and is the primary way that endurance exercise improves the heart. It becomes bigger and capable of delivering more blood per beat to all the waiting muscles of the body.

At rest an untrained person's heart may put out about 2 ounces per beat with about 70 beats per minute. That yields an output of 140 ounces—a little more than one gallon per minute. If this same person endurance-trains for three months, the resting heart rate may decrease to 55 beats per minute while the per-stroke volume could rise to 2.5 ounces. That would yield about the same output as before—just more than a gallon per minute at rest.

So the fit athlete's submaximal heart rate is lower than when he or she was unfit. In highly fit endurance athletes the resting heart rate per minute may be in the 30s or low 40s. Such low heart rates mean a large stroke volume and are an indicator of increasing fitness.

[The Plumbing]

The heart is a little larger than your fist, weighs a bit less than a pound, and is situated about in the center of your chest just beneath the breastbone and between the lungs. It is actually made up of two side-by-side pumps. The right side pumps blood through the pulmonary artery to the lungs, where it picks up oxygen and gives off carbon dioxide before returning by way of the pulmonary vein to the heart's left atrium. The left side pump sends the oxygen-rich blood to the rest of the body through the aorta and arterial network. The blood returns to the right side of the heart by way of the veins, and the process starts all over again. Each side of the heart has a thin-walled receiving chamber (the atrium) that helps to fill the thick-walled major pump (the ventricle). One-way valves separate the atria from the ventricles to prevent backflow. Similar valves at the exits of the atria keep the blood flowing in the right directions.

Figure 2.1 shows blood flow through the heart. Notice the size of the left ventricle compared with the right one. Pumping blood to the exercising body takes more force than pumping it to the lungs, making the left ventricle larger.

Your body contains about a gallon of blood, which makes up roughly 8 pounds of your body weight, depending on your body size. This blood is continuously recirculated. Each day, your heart beats about 100,000 times and pumps something like 5,000 gallons of blood.

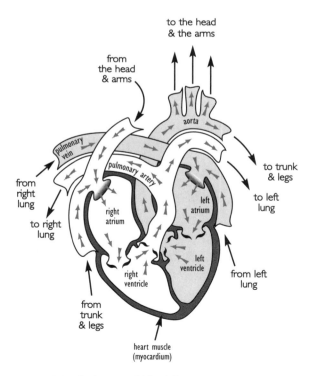

Figure 2.1. The heart and blood flow

[The Spark Plug]

Just as the engine in your car has a spark plug, the heart has special electrical cells to stimulate it to beat. This natural spark plug is in the upper part of the right atrium and is known as the sinus node. When you step on the gas pedal in your car the spark plugs fire faster to generate a greater number of sparks per minute. In terms of the heart, the gas pedal is the hormone commonly called adrenaline, which causes the sinus node to increase the number of sparks per minute. A network of nerves conducts the spark all over the heart, and this causes contraction of the atria and ventricles to pump the blood. Your heart rate monitor chest strap senses this electrical activity and transmits the data to your receiver.

THE ATHLETE'S HEART

The endurance athlete's heart differs from the nonathlete's mostly in size. The heart of the athlete is a bit larger, primarily because of the increased capacity of the left ventricle. For many years this was considered to be unhealthy because such sizes often bordered on being pathologic. Today, however, cardiologists can differentiate between the athletic and pathologically enlarged hearts and recognize that the athlete's bigger heart is not unhealthy and is, in fact, just the opposite.

Nevertheless, seemingly fit athletes do die during exercise. About 100 people die each year in the United States while engaged in sport. Nearly all of them have some form of heart disease. Being fit is not the same as being healthy. A good example of this is the untimely death of Jim Fixx in 1984.

Fixx was the author of *The Complete Book of Running* (Random House, 1977), the best-selling, nonfiction hardcover book ever published by that time, which helped to create the running boom and benefited from it. It was in this book that Fixx said if you ran a marathon you would never die of heart disease. On July 20, 1984, at age 52, he died while on a 10-mile run in Vermont, having trained for 17 years and completed 20 marathons. An autopsy revealed blockage in Fixx's three main heart arteries of up to 95 percent. It was apparently genetic, as his father had experienced a heart attack at age 35 and 7 years later died during a second such incident. Regardless of how fit you may consider yourself, it's a good idea to have periodic checkups by your doctor. Things do go wrong—even with athletes' hearts.

There is no doubt, though, that the healthy athlete's heart is not the norm for our society. Chronic exercise produces changes in the heart, changes that make it stronger and more effective. Heart rate is also affected by exercise. Here are some things you might expect to see in your heart rate as a result of exercise.

[Resting Heart Rate]

Your heart rate while fully relaxed and sitting or lying down is your resting heart rate (RHR) and is a decent indicator of changes in cardiovascular fitness. A gradual decline in RHR over several weeks is a fairly accurate predictor of improving cardiovascular fitness and probably indicates that the heart's blood pumped per beat, called "stroke volume," is increasing and that the muscles are more efficient at removing oxygen from the blood.

Normally, the RHR is 15 to 20 beats per minute lower than your daily heart rate when you're standing and walking around. For fit endurance athletes, RHR is generally in the range of 40 to 60, but it is not unusual to find athletes with an RHR in the 30s. The lowest RHR recorded in the scientific literature was 28. Sedentary people generally have an RHR in the range of 60 to 80 but exceeds 100 in a few. Research has generally shown a positive correlation between RHR and the risk of cardiovascular disease—that is, the lower the RHR, the lower the risk.

But be careful about what you read into your RHR. A low RHR should not be taken as a sure sign that you don't have something wrong with your heart. In the same way, a comparatively high (for endurance athletes) RHR is not necessarily a sign that you are in poor aerobic condition. Jim Ryun, the great American miler of the 1970s, is reported to have had an RHR in the low 70s even when in peak form, a ridiculously high RHR for a world-class endurance athlete. Heredity plays a role in RHR.

Later I'll show you how to use RHR to monitor your adaptive state—how well your body is coping with the stresses of training and life in general. It's a good idea to start building a record of your RHR as you read this book over the next few days. To do this, put your heart rate monitor on the nightstand next to your bed. When you wake up in the morning, slowly put it on and then lie back down for 5 minutes. Watch your heart rate drop and record in your training log the lowest number you observe. You'll find that it varies a bit from day to day, as a result of both the physical and psychological stress you're experiencing at the time.

[Exercise Response]

Heart rate is regulated by the autonomic nervous system. During rest the parasympathetic branch of the system keeps heart rate low. As soon as you start any activity, including standing up after sitting for a few minutes reading this book, the sympathetic branch kicks in and elevates heart rate by causing the release of adrenaline, which stimulates the sinus node in the right atrium to increase the rate at which its spark is delivered to the heart muscle. The sympathetic nervous system also boosts breathing rate and blood pressure as vigorous exercise begins.

During exercise, the amount of blood pumped by the heart must increase to match the increased demand of the working muscles. It regulates this by matching heart rate to demand through a feedback loop. That is, the more intensely you exercise, the higher your heart rate goes. This is why we use a heart rate monitor to help gauge the intensity of exercise, and thus our heart rate. But just as with RHR, as your aerobic fitness develops, your body's muscles' ability to pull oxygen out of the blood improves, and so your heart rate decreases at any given level of work output (pace or power) below the maximum. This drop in exercise heart rate is another good indicator of improving aerobic fitness. In Chapter 4 I'll show you a simple way to use this phenomenon to test and measure changes in fitness.

Early in a workout your heart rate responds more slowly to increases in intensity than it does late in the workout. This is most noticeable when doing high-intensity intervals after a short warm-up. For the first minute or two of the first interval, heart rate rises slowly, so you must gauge how hard to go based on perceived exertion, pace, or power. As the workout progresses, however, your heart beats faster earlier in the interval. For very short intervals, of about 30 seconds or less, this slowness to respond simply means that heart rate by itself is not a good way to regulate intensity.

[Maximum Heart Rate]

The maximum heart rate (MHR) is the highest number of beats per minute for your heart. While many coaches and athletes believe this is the most important of all your heart rate data, I disagree and will explain why in Chapter 3. It's an interesting number, but not necessarily the critical one for understanding how to use your heart rate monitor to the greatest effect.

Just as with all heart rate data, MHR is specific to sport. For example, a triathlete would find that her MHR is *not* the same for swimming, biking, and running. It is generally highest for running and lowest for swimming. This has to do with the amount of muscle mass being used to propel the body, as well as other factors such as vertical versus horizontal body postures and the effects in the pool of gravity and buoyancy.

Trying to find your MHR is a daunting task. I do not recommend it. Doing so requires gun-to-the-head motivation and an extreme effort for several minutes, often repeated as in an interval workout. If you are even a bit tired from previous training, the chances are good you will come up well short of your actual MHR.

Such field testing also isn't safe for many athletes. If you decide to try it, speak with your doctor first if you are over age 35, have a family history of heart disease, are overweight, have been sedentary for a number of years, or are in poor physical condition. *Do not take MHR testing lightly.* You are better off not trying to find your MHR regardless of how healthy and fit you are. There just isn't a compelling reason to do so.

[Recovery Heart Rate]

The recovery heart rate occurs in two phases. One is the first minute after exercise, during which heart rate drops rapidly, and the other is the longer recovery plateau, during which the heart rate decreases slowly. The plateau phase may last from 30 minutes to several hours, depending on the preceding workout and your level of fitness. The difference between your workout-ending heart rate and 1-minute recovery heart rate is what we are interested in here.

Your recovery heart rate differential (RHRD) is found by subtracting your heart rate 1 minute after stopping exercise from your heart rate at the time you stopped. RHRD generally increases as your fitness improves. It is specific to the intensity and duration of the preceding workout. Long workouts tend to produce lower RHRD than short ones. Highly intense workouts result in greater RHRD than easy ones. After taking all this into consideration, keeping tabs on your RHRD tells you with some degree of certainty how your physical fitness is progressing.

It may also say something about your cardiac health. In a study reported in the *New England Journal of Medicine* in 1999, the authors reported a strong correlation between RHRD and the risk of heart attack. They followed 2,400 patients for about six years, during which time 213 of them died. Simply determining RHRD was a better predictor of mortality than commonly accepted and much more expensive medical tests that measure blood flow to and electrical activity of the heart. People with a low RHRD—less than 20—were the ones who were at high risk for death from heart disease.

[Cardiac Drift]

During extended exercise your heart rate is likely to gradually rise, even though your work output measured as a pace or power remains constant. You may have started the workout with a heart rate of 135 and two hours later it is at 150 although your pace or power has not changed at all. This is known as "cardiac drift" and is not fully understood. In extreme cases heart rate can drift upward by perhaps as much as 25 beats per minute after an hour of exercise. What this means for your training and racing is that if you are gauging intensity based strictly on heart rate, any attempt to maintain a constant heart rate will result in a gradual slowing down of your activity.

Cardiac drift is most likely the result of a rise in the body's core temperature combined with the onset of dehydration, since it is most evident in hot-weather exercise. Dehydration decreases all body fluids, including the water in your blood. As the blood becomes thicker it becomes harder to pump, causing the heart to work harder. So there is a gradual increase in heart rate. One study found a 7-beat-per-minute increase for each 1 percent of body weight loss caused by dehydration. Weight losses of 3 to even 4 percent are common in hot weather during extensive exercise.

Another possible cause is fatigue. During a long, hard workout some of your muscles grow tired and no longer are able to keep going. So the brain compensates by calling on other muscles in the region to work harder. These muscles may not be positioned as well to do the work, or they may be better suited for powerful contractions rather than endurance work. In either case the heart will have to pump faster to deliver blood to these less-effective muscles. So heart rate increases.

As an athlete's aerobic fitness improves, cardiac drift declines. Even in very hot conditions a fit athlete will experience only minor upticks in heart rate. For example, I coach an Ironman triathlete who lives in the Phoenix area. Early in the summer, when his fitness and heat adaptation are improving but still marginal, we have seen very high cardiac drift rates relative to his running pace or bike power. But by the end of the summer, even with temperatures mounting to the low 100s, we see only minor drifting—as little as 1 percent during a five-hour, steady-state bike ride.

In Chapter 4 I'll show you how to use cardiac drift as a standard to measure changes in aerobic fitness.

WHAT AFFECTS YOUR HEART RATE?

Besides cardiac drift, you can expect many other factors to influence your heart rate. Understanding these will help you to prevent those that are avoidable and so train more precisely.

[Daily Variations]

Research has shown day-to-day variations in heart rate of 2 to 6 beats per minute at the same workload. This is because we are humans and not machines. You probably know that you experience minor changes in stress and recovery even when everything is going well and you are well rested. Minor variations in heart rate–based test or workout results, either positive or negative, should not be assumed to be anything more than your humanity at work.

You should always strive to recover quickly after workouts. Consistently high heart rates, even on days of easy workouts, are a sign that you aren't recovering well. You're either over-training or not paying close enough attention to those factors that speed recovery—rest and diet. In *The Paleo Diet for Athletes,* Loren Cordain, Ph.D., and I describe how to modify your nutrition for rapid recovery.

[Body Temperature]

As mentioned above, a rise in body tempera-ture, which is to be expected during exercise regardless of intensity or other conditions, causes an increase in heart rate. The higher your tem-perature rises, the more your heart rate is also likely to increase. Strategies to keep body tem-perature under control in hot weather include clothing selection, time of day for workout, pac-ing modification, and liberal use of ice.

[Gravity]

The effect of gravity, or lack thereof, affects your heart rate. This is most evident in water. For example, an injured runner will often go to a deep swimming pool to run without stressing the injury. What becomes immediately obvious when doing this is that heart rate does not rise nearly as fast as it does when running on dry land. When the body is buoyant, there is little vertical movement as when pounding the pave-ment. Overcoming the restraints of gravity requires a considerable amount of effort. When gravity is reduced by running in water, it takes a gargantuan effort to produce the same heart rates as were experienced out on the roads with only a moderate effort.

On dry land, gravity favors a pooling of blood in the legs, forcing the heart to work harder to move it around the entire body. This also results in an elevated heart rate.

By contrast, gravity can be your best friend when training to improve fitness. That's why hill training is so effective.

[Position]

In sports such as cycling, body position and pos-ture can both affect heart rate. One study of elite cyclists found that although the use of aerodynamic handlebars on a racing bicycle cre-ated a streamlined position that maximized per-formance, it also caused a rise in heart rate of 5 beats per minute when riding at 70 percent of aerobic capacity compared with a more upright position. This may be due to a less-efficient hip angle. But, intriguingly, many cyclists and triath-letes report that the lower, bent-over position produces lower heart rates than does sitting

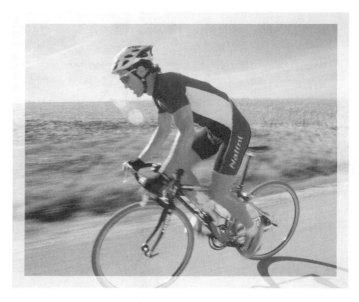

upright. More research is needed, it seems. Fine-tuning a cyclist's bike fit may well keep heart rate in check, but a poor position may magnify it.

[Heat]

HR tends to be lower in cold weather and higher in hot weather at the same effort. The difference could be as much as 10 to 30 beats per minute. So heart rate is a less reliable measure of exercise intensity in the heat, but it does accurately reflect the stress the body is experiencing. Once heart rate is elevated owing to heat, even when the workload is reduced heart rate remains high. So on hot days it's best to start the workout or the race at a somewhat conservative workload.

How much you need to back off depends on how hot it is, how well adapted you are, and the nature of your sport. It takes about two weeks of exposure to high temperatures during workouts to fully adapt. Heat adaptation results in lower skin temperatures, higher sweat rates, and lower heart rates. Although somewhat reduced, heat stress remains a challenge even for the well adapted. The reason heart rate increases under hot conditions is attributable to the body's way of cooling itself. When body temperature begins to rise above normal levels, more blood is sent to the skin to give off heat, much as the radiator in your car works to cool the engine. If the muscles are also demanding blood to maintain a high work level during exercise, the heart has no choice but to speed up its pumping. Thus your heart rate rises.

Your sport may also play a role in how hot it feels during exercise. As a result of the greater movement of air over the body (and thus evaporation), an athlete in high-velocity sports such as cycling or rowing is likely to experience less heat stress than a runner, given the same conditions.

Some research studies conducted at temperatures just above freezing have shown heart rate to decrease during exercise for men but not for women when both were lightly clad. Not all studies have found this gender difference, however, nor have they all found lower heart rates in the cold. So the jury is still out on this one.

[Humidity]

High humidity has the same effect on heart rate as high air temperatures, and for the same reason: The heart is working hard to cool the body and fuel the muscles.

[Equipment]

The equipment you use may also affect your heart rate. You will work harder with a higher heart rate if your gear is heavy, fits poorly, or is not aerodynamic or hydrodynamic. For example, a runner wearing heavy training shoes will have a slightly higher heart rate than if he were wearing lightweight racing flats and running at the same pace. But realize that there is always a trade-off when it comes to light equipment. It tends to cost more and not last as long as heavier gear.

[Technique]

Inefficient technique wastes a tremendous amount of energy, which is always associated with high heart rates. A runner who bounces up and down excessively, a swimmer who "fishtails," and a cyclist who sways from side to side while mashing the pedals will work harder than necessary at any given pace or power. The highly efficient athlete makes the movements of the sport look easy, wastes little energy, and keeps heart rate in check.

Technique is the area in which most amateur endurance athletes have the greatest room for improvement, yet few of them work on skills. Many incorrectly consider their sport to be non-skilled. Or they believe that whatever technique they use just happens to be what they were born with, and messing with it will only make them less efficient. I've even heard coaches say this. The truth is that skills for all endurance sports *can* be improved and training to do so *will* eventually result in lower heart rates at any given workload and significant performance gains.

[Caffeine]

Scientific studies of the effects of caffeine on heart rate have produced mixed results. Several have shown an increased heart rate during exercise at a fixed workload after the ingestion of caffeine, while others have found no change. One study reported that in the first few minutes of exercise there was a drop in heart rate below the baseline, followed later by an increase above it. Many of these studies were done with people who generally avoid caffeine, but others were done with regular caffeine users. While the preponderance of evidence seems to indicate that caffeine increases heart rate during exercise, the facts are just not in. There may be individual differences.

[Drugs]

Both over-the-counter and prescription drugs are likely to affect heart rate. Some drugs, such as diuretics, have been shown to decrease heart rate while others, like cold remedies, are likely to raise it. How much depends on many factors, such as your age, weight, physical condition, and, of course, type of drug and dosage. Some medications may also cause arrhythmias. When taking some drugs it is best that you not exercise at all. Before taking *any* drug, it is a good idea to talk with your doctor about how wise it is to exercise and what the drug's side effects might be.

[Altitude]

If you go to a high-altitude place to race or train, your heart rate will be higher for a given pace or power. While this will be moderated somewhat after two weeks or so of adaptation to altitude, heart rate will still be somewhat higher than if you were at sea level doing the same workout. In the first couple of weeks in a place like Colorado it's best to reduce your training volume to allow your body to adjust without undue additional stress.

Since high altitude tends to cause a decrease in muscular force because of reduced oxygen intake, you won't be able to go as fast as you would under the same conditions at a low altitude. So while you may experience increased levels of red blood cells and improved cardiovascular fitness as a result of high-altitude exposure, you may see a decrease in the fitness of the overall muscular system. To counteract this, when I coach athletes who live or train at altitude, I have them do lots of short intervals, generally less than 2 minutes long, with recoveries that are longer than the work intervals. Short hill repeats are also effective for maintaining the muscular systems of runners, cyclists, and cross-country skiers.

[Emotion]

Your hormonal levels can affect heart rate. Anxiety or nervousness before a race will cause

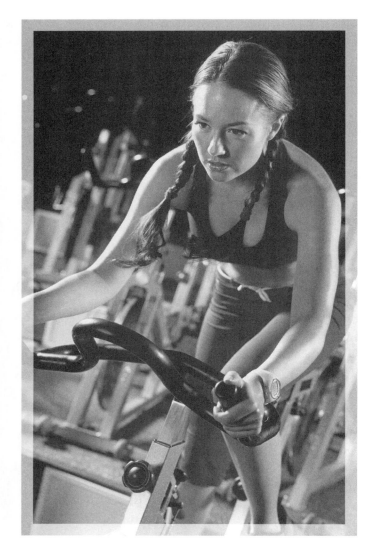

Before races it is a good idea to calm yourself down as much as possible to prevent going out too fast early in the race and then fading fast later on. Your heart rate monitor is one of the best tools there is for controlling prerace anxiety. By paying close attention to your heart rate in the hours and minutes leading up to a competition, you can control your level of arousal, allowing you to start at a much wiser intensity.

[Age]

It appears, based on most research, that as we age our maximal heart rate declines but that there is no change in our resting heart rate. That's certainly true of our sedentary neighbors, but not necessarily true for athletes. The research is not in agreement when it comes to very active people. For example, one study that compared masters in their late 50s and early 60s with young athletes in their 20s found that the older athletes' maximal heart rates were 14 percent lower. The two groups of athletes were matched based on how similarly they trained. Another study, however, conducted over eight years found no change in max heart rates of endurance athletes by their early 60s, while the sedentary age-matched group experienced an 8-beat-per-minute decline.

the release of adrenaline from the adrenal gland, which all by itself elevates your heart rate. This is a result of your evolutionary survival reflex known as the fight–flight reaction. It helped to save your Paleolithic ancestors from sabertooth cats. Today it is still there to "protect" you from the competition in your race category. You may experience the same phenomenon when under psychological stress of any kind.

Anecdotally, I have found no loss of max heart rates in older athletes I have coached who have been training at a high level for decades. My own top-end heart rate on the bike has been 172 for the last 23 years that I have been observing it with a wireless heart rate monitor, and I am age 62 as of this writing. Despite my experience and study, I can't explain why much of the research disagrees with what I have seen.

It may have to do with how strenuously an athlete trains in the face of advancing age.

Other research has shown that stroke volume—the amount of blood pumped per heart beat—does not decline in aging athletes and that heart size remains about the same if training intensity is maintained over time. The aging athlete's heart is considerably larger, with a greater stroke volume, than that of her sedentary age mates. So any changes in heart rate due to aging are probably not related to heart size or contractility. That leaves the nervous system and the sinus node (the "spark plug") as the likely causes of declines in max heart rate with aging.

Aging appears to also reduce the elasticity of the arteries, even with continued and challenging workouts. You can get a sense of this loss of elasticity by pulling the skin on the back of your hand and watching how quickly it returns to normal when released. In young people the skin snaps back like a rubber band. In older people it seems to "ooze" back. Your arteries are doing much the same thing. As a result of this "hardening" of the arteries, blood pressure rises gradually by perhaps 0.5 percent per year. For the older athlete, this results in an increased arterial resistance to blood flow, since the arteries don't stretch and contract as easily with each beat of the heart, meaning that the heart must work harder to overcome the resistance. At low intensity, however, the small decrease in blood flow due to the aging plumbing is compensated for by aging athletes' increased ability to pull oxygen out of the blood at the working muscle.

[Gender Differences]

Women tend to have slightly higher heart rates than men, simply because they often are small-er. This means they also have somewhat smaller hearts. Since the heart is smaller, it pumps less blood per beat and therefore has to beat faster than a man's to deliver oxygen and fuel to the muscles at the same workload.

[Cadence]

The cadence with which you run, pedal, swim, or row at affects your heart rate. Let's do a "mental research study" to better understand this. If you took the chain off a bike and pedaled it at a very slow cadence, such as 40 revolutions per minute (RPM), and then at a very high cadence, such as 100 RPM, would you notice a difference in your heart rate? Most certainly. Even though the power applied to the rear wheel is zero in both cases, the heart beats faster at a higher RPM. Therefore, cadence, or the rhythmical measure of activity or motion, and heart rate are closely linked, regardless of sport.

Now, don't take this to mean that you should use the lowest possible cadence for your sport. That's seldom beneficial to performance. As RPM decrease, the demand on the individual muscles increases. As RPM increase, assuming the same workload (power or pace), the aerobic system is increasingly challenged as the muscles experience less load. In other words, at low RPM you feel the work primarily in your legs or arms, while at high RPM you feel it in your breathing. The trick is to find just the right balance between the stress felt both in the arms or legs and in the lungs. When you find this balance point, you are at your most efficient cadence.

It's possible to change this most economical cadence through training. When you first try exercising at a new cadence, you will be uneconomical, meaning you will waste more energy than usual. But over time as your body adapts, especially your nervous and muscular systems, the new cadence will become increasingly economical.

[Time of Day]

Many of the physiological responses to exercise vary by time of day. Heart rate is no different. It tends to be lower during submaximal exercise done in the morning compared with the afternoon. And this tendency has been shown to increase with age. So it appears that as you get older you are more likely to become a "morning person." The difference in morning versus afternoon exercise heart rates is rather small but can be significant, on the order of 3 to 8 beats per minute.

[Dehydration]

During intense exercise in hot or humid conditions, you can lose more than a quart of body fluids in an hour, mostly due to sweating. As fluid is lost there is a decrease in blood plasma, making the blood more viscous. "Thicker" blood means the heart must work harder by contracting faster to pump it. Heart rate could easily rise 10 to 30 beats per minute with dehydration. An unusually high heart rate during exercise may well be a sign that you are dehydrating and need to take in more fluids.

[Illness]

When you are sick, your heart rate may be elevated. Some types of infection raise the heart rate, since the body is working hard to fight off an invader. But heart rate is probably not the best indicator that something is wrong. How you feel is still the main way to determine if you

are in the early stages of catching a bug. Your resting heart rate may simply help to confirm this.

HEART RATE MISCONCEPTIONS

When it comes to heart rate, athletes and people in general have many mistaken beliefs. Some of these are even propagated by well-studied and well-meaning professionals such as doctors, exercise scientists, physical trainers, and coaches. Here are three common heart rate misconceptions.

[Misconception 1: Max Heart Rate = 220 – Age]

The formula above is as likely to be wrong— way wrong!—as it is to be right. In sport science, where a reliability quotient of 0.95 is considered good, this formula's reliability is 0.51. In other words, it's reliable only about half the time. And yet exercise physiology textbooks continue to quote it as if it were the gospel. Your family doctor probably uses it to estimate your heart rate, and if you are tested in a clinic they also will predict your maximum heart rate from this formula. Gyms and aerobics rooms across the country have posters on the wall based on 220 – age.

This old formula grew out of a 1971 review of the scientific literature on the topic of the relationship between physical activity and heart rate by Fox and colleagues. Interestingly, the paper cites only 35 data points to support the formula and concludes that the margin of error is "not far from many of the data points." A subsequent review of the same literature in 2002 showed that predicting heart rate from those same 35 data points would result in an error of at least 21 beats too high or too low—a massive swing of 42 beats per minute (bpm)!

Newer formulas have done somewhat better, but are still well off the mark. For example, the formula

$$208.754 - 0.734 \times age$$

has been shown to have an error of about plus or minus 7.2 bpm. A bit more accurate is the even newer formula

$$205.8 - 0.685 \times age$$

which has proved to be off 6.4 bpm high or low. But don't count on them even being that close. For example, both formulas produce about the same predicted max heart rate for me—163.2 and 163.3. For cycling they are about 9 beats per minute low and for running about 17 beats low.

There is currently no fool-proof way to estimate max heart rate because there are simply too many variables like those described above, such as age, gender, fitness, health, and mode of exercise used. The only way to know your maximum heart rate is to exercise to your maximum capacity wearing a heart rate monitor. But that isn't recommended either. The only reason you might even want to know this number is to set up your heart rate training zones. We have less stressful and more accurate ways to do that, which will be described in Chapter 3. So let's move beyond max heart rate concerns.

[Misconception 2: To Lose Weight, Exercise in the "Fat Burning Zone"]

The myth of the "fat-burning zone" has been around for a few decades now, and, like most myths, it has an element of truth to it. It's true that when you exercise at a low intensity your primary source of fuel is fat. So why isn't going slow always the best way to shed blubber? Let's examine what happens during exercise.

The body has two primary sources of fuel to use during exercise—fat and glycogen. Glycogen is a form of carbohydrate stored in the muscles. During aerobic activity both glycogen and fat are used simultaneously to provide energy. At low intensity a greater percentage of the fuel comes from fat, but some of the energy is also supplied by glycogen. As the intensity of exercise increases—for example, going from walking to running—the body gradually begins to use more glycogen and less fat. At very high intensities, such as long sprints, most of the energy is supplied by glycogen, with relatively little coming from fat.

Still sounds like slow exercise is the way to go, right? Read on.

The confounding factor has to do with how many total calories are burned during low-intensity and high-intensity exercise. When you are going slow, fewer calories are used per unit of time than when going fast.

Let's say, for example, that there are two 150-pound people, each with 30 minutes to exercise. One walks and the other runs. Our walker covers 2 miles and burns about 200 calories. Of these, 70 percent came from fat, for a total of 140 fat calories used. The runner covers 3 miles in the same 30 minutes and consumes 330 calories, with 60 percent of them derived from fat—198 calories.

The higher-intensity exercise increased the amount fat burned by more than 40 percent.

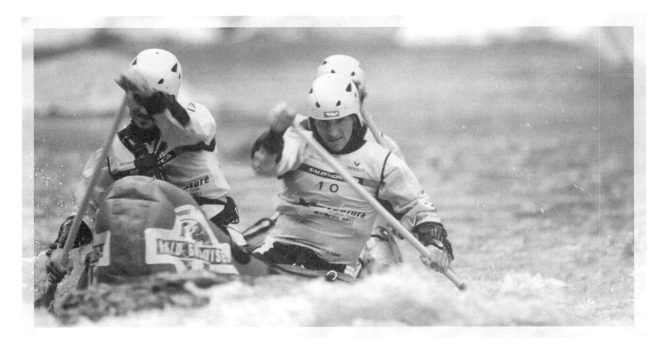

What it comes down to is this: Do you want a big slice of a little pie, or a small slice of a big pie? While you'll usually take pie any way you can get it, the bigger pie (the higher-intensity workout) is definitely better for burning fat.

And there's more. For some time after the workout, perhaps a few minutes to a few hours, your metabolism is elevated above baseline levels. Suet is melting away even though you are sitting at your desk. The higher the intensity and the greater duration of the workout, the higher the metabolism and the more calories that are burned. When it comes to counting calories, high intensity results in more calories expended than staying in the so-called fat-burning zone.

That doesn't mean you should always exercise intensely. When starting an exercise program, going slowly reduces the risk of injury. Also, easy exercise days are needed after hard days, to allow muscles and other systems to recover.

[Misconception 3: The Purpose of Training Is to Increase Heart Rate]

I'm afraid that some athletes have lost track of what training is all about since they got heart rate monitors. They seem to believe that the purpose of training is to make their hearts beat faster. Over time they want to see higher heart rates when they work out, and they take that as a sign of improved fitness. Unfortunately, they've got it backward. The purpose of training is to get more output (power or pace) for the same input (heart rate). At the finish of a race they don't give awards to those who recorded the highest heart rates. The prizes go to those who were fastest.

What you would actually like to see happen to heart rate is that it gets lower over time. Or that you get faster at the same heart rate. This is what training is all about, and it's quite measurable using your heart rate monitor. For example, one way to determine an improvement in fitness is to cover a fixed distance at a standard heart rate. If your time improves even though heart rate and effort both stay the same, then your fitness is also improving.

THE HEART OF THE MATTER

The athlete's heart is a complex device with an incredible capacity for change—for better or worse. When used strenuously, as during endurance exercise, it grows stronger and capable of delivering huge amounts of blood to the working muscles. When not stressed, it loses functional capacity and is susceptible to disease.

The positive and measurable changes in heart rate due to chronic exercise are a reduction in resting heart rate and heart rate at any given level of intensity, and an increase in the rate at which the heart rate falls in the first minute after exercise.

Heart rate from maximal to recovery is specific to the sport. You cannot assume that if you know how your heart responds to exercise in one sport, you therefore know how your heart responds to *all* sports. This is most critical for the triathlete who must get to know her heart rate for each of three sports.

The duration of the workout affects heart rate, which tends to rise in the later stages even if the pace or power stays the same. This is called cardiac drift. As fitness improves, cardiac drift decreases under the same conditions. Other factors that affect your exercising heart rate are how rested you are, body temperature, gravity, position or posture, heat and humidity, equipment used, technique, caffeine, drugs, altitude, emotion, age, gender, cadence, time of day, dehydration, and illness.

Three common misconceptions about heart rate are that max heart rate may be found by subtracting your age from 220, that low-heart-rate exercise is best for burning body fat, and that the purpose of training is to increase heart rate.

3

GETTING
STARTED

Having a good heart rate monitor and understanding how it and your heart work isn't enough. You must also understand how heart rate can be used as a tool to make your exercise more purposeful and effective. In this chapter you will learn how to determine and use heart rate zones to give your training focus and clarity.

MONITORING INTENSITY

Whether you are an Olympic medalist, a back-of-the-packer hoping to finish, or just someone serious about exercise, you need to know the only four things you can change in training to improve your fitness—mode, frequency, duration, and intensity. It's the same for everyone, whether a green novice or a grizzled veteran or a young Olympian. To fully grasp heart rate training, you need to have a good understanding of these basics.

Mode is the method of exercise you choose for a workout. A runner runs and a swimmer swims. A triathlete swims, then rides a bike, and finally runs. Each of these is a mode. Modes that are the same as the competitions you do are "specific" modes. Nonspecific modes are called "general" training. They are also sometimes referred to as "cross training." When a runner lifts weights, she is cross training. There are times in the season when you will want to cross train and others when you will use only a specific mode. This is explained in Chapter 7.

Frequency refers to how often you work out in a given period of time, usually a week. You may do 1 workout each day for a frequency of 7, or do 2-a-days for a frequency of 14.

Duration simply has to do with how long your workouts are. Your workouts may have a duration of 40 minutes or 4 hours. Generally, workout durations vary throughout the week, based on your purpose for each session.

When frequency and duration are combined, we call the result *volume*. So if you have a frequency of 6 and each workout's duration is 30 minutes, your volume is 3 hours. Or this could be expressed in accumulated distance covered. You're probably used to talking about volume in this way. When someone asks how much you are running (or whatever your sport is), you may say 30 miles per week. Either way, that's volume you're describing.

Mode, frequency, duration, and volume are easy to describe. *Intensity* is a bit of a challenge and, in fact, we have no commonly accepted way of describing accumulated intensity for a week, as we do with volume. It can even be difficult to describe intensity for a single workout. Yet, interestingly, the scientific literature tells us without exception that the intensity of training is the most important element. So it's curious that we lack at least several methods for describing it, regardless of sport. The following is a brief look at some of the ways intensity is typically described and measured. These may vary a bit, from sport to sport. But as you'll see, one that does cut across all sports is heart rate.

[Rating of Perceived Exertion]

Perhaps the oldest and most common way to explain intensity is to simply rate how hard a workout is, using everyday language. You could, for example, say that your workout is very easy or moderately hard. The problem with this is that the person you are talking with may not interpret your words as intended. So out of this confusion grew a numeric, exercise-intensity rating system. There have been various versions created. The easiest for most athletes to learn and use is the 1-to-10 scale.

On such a scale 1 represents an extremely easy effort—as easy as you could possibly exercise—and 10 the hardest possible effort. The next time you work out, try assigning a number to how difficult you are exercising at that moment. This is your Rating of Perceived Exertion (RPE). Get used to rating your effort as you train this way. It's a useful tool that you will soon learn to use in conjunction with heart rate. Table 3.1 summarizes the details of RPE.

VELOCITY

Another well-established system for defining intensity is velocity—how fast you are moving. For running and cross-country skiing, velocity is usually expressed as pace—minutes per mile or per kilometer. Swimmers also generally refer to velocity as pace, only it's as time per 100 meters or yards. In cycling, velocity is described as speed—miles or kilometers per hour. All of these are a fairly accurate system as long as the course is flat and wind or rough water is not an issue. If they are an issue, then workout or race intensities are not easily compared.

POWER

As a way of expressing exercise intensity in watts, power is relatively new. Cycling and indoor rowing are the two endurance sports in which the concept of power is becoming increasingly popular. Some running treadmills

RPE	LEVEL OF EXERTION	BREATHING
1	Extremely easy	Restful breathing, can sing
2	Very easy	Can talk in complete sentences
3	Easy	Can talk in broken sentences
4	Moderate	Talking first becomes difficult
5	Somewhat hard	Heavy breathing begins
6	Moderately hard	Deep breaths, talking is avoided
7	Hard	Deep and forceful breathing
8	Very hard	Labored, cannot talk
9	Very, very hard	Very labored breathing
10	Extremely hard	Gasping for air

Table 3.1. Rating of Perceived Exertion

also display power. This is a highly accurate method of indicating intensity, since the typical confounding factors of diet, weather, and terrain have no effect on power. The downside of power, however, is that it relies heavily on a high technology, making powermeters expensive compared with other intensity-measuring systems. For example, the least expensive bicycle powermeter retails for about 10 times the cost of a basic heart rate monitor.

LACTATE ACCUMULATION

To understand this measure of intensity, we need to start with a little biochemistry. As your body uses carbohydrate to create energy, it releases a by-product inside the muscle cell called lactic acid. This soon begins to seep out of the muscle cell into the surrounding space and bloodstream and in doing so changes its composition by giving off hydrogen ions. This hydrogen, not the lactate, is what causes the burning sensation in your muscles at high effort levels. Despite its "bad boy" reputation, lactate is actually a beneficial substance for the body during exercise, as it is used by the body to create more energy so that exercise may continue. It's the hydrogen that is the real acidic culprit. But measuring the lactate levels in the blood is a convenient way of estimating how much acid is in the body. The more intense the workout, the greater the amount of lactate released into the blood—and thus the more hydrogen ions.

Until the late 1990s measuring lactate was a lab-only activity. But then less-expensive and even portable lactate analyzers began to appear on the market. With one of these devices an athlete could draw blood samples from a finger or earlobe after each interval in a workout,

measure the lactate, and decide whether the intensity needed adjusting on the next interval. Lactate is also a good way to gauge progress in periodic testing. If, over the course of a few weeks, lactate levels fall relative to the workload in a standard test, then we can assume that fitness has improved.

The obvious downsides of lactate measurement are that it requires drawing blood and that the sampling methodology is rather delicate. It is best to have a well-trained technician do the sampling rather than doing it yourself. This is not the best intensity-monitoring system for most athletes.

HEART RATE

Monitoring heart rate has proven to be an effective way to gauge the intensity of a workout. What we are actually measuring with a heart rate monitor is the body's response to the demands of your workout. Since a higher RPE means the muscles need an increased supply of oxygen and nutrients to produce energy, the heart must beat faster to meet the demand. So there is a close correlation between intensity and heart rate. Typically, as the intensity (or RPE) rises, heart rate also rises.

To make sense of the numbers, heart rate training zones are needed to define how hard the workout is. These zones vary by sport, because the heart response is unique for each type of exercise. The biggest variables are gravity and the amount of muscle required by the sport. So running, which has a slight vertical component and therefore a significant gravity demand and uses nearly all the big, lower-body muscles, produces high heart rate zones. By contrast, swimming has a low gravity demand since the athlete is buoyant and most of the muscle used for propulsion is in the upper body, where the muscles are smaller than those of the legs.

There are always exceptions, however. Well-conditioned and competitive swimmers often report seeing higher heart rates in the pool than when running. This may be due in part to their greater capacity for work when swimming than when running.

While the absolute heart rates seen may be higher in a sport like running than in swimming, the RPE stays the same. For example, a triathlete who runs with an RPE of 7 and a heart rate of 160 bpm feels the same as when swimming at a 7 RPE even though his heart rate may now be 145. Using heart rate training zones helps to make sense of this, so long as the zones are set up relative to each sport. In other words, you can't use the same zone numbers for all sports.

LT—THE HEART OF TRAINING

To set up your heart rate zones, we must have a reference point. The most common way to do this, although not the best, is to determine your maximum heart rate. This is usually done by subtracting your age from 220. Don't use this method, because it's as likely to be wrong as right. This formula is really only good for talking about large groups of people—not individuals.

For example, if we could determine the actual maximum heart rates for everyone who lives in a city by testing and then graphing the results, based on the relationship between their ages and their max heart rates as predicted by the formula, we'd create a bell-shaped curve. We'd see that most of the subjects fall into the

middle of the curve. For these people the formula is pretty good at predicting max heart rate. But for those on either end of the curve the prediction is either too high or low. It could be off by more than 20 beats per minute either way. That's huge. Since we don't know where you fall on the curve, we're likely to have your reference heart rate way off. That would make your heart rate zones inaccurate and thus useless.

Another common way to determine actual, rather than estimated, max heart rate is to have the athlete complete a series of short, all-out efforts, trying to drive his heart rate as high as possible by about the third repetition. That is likely to be very close to max heart rate if the athlete is highly motivated. If motivation is lacking, the test results are of little value.

But let's assume that you are highly motivated that day and come up with an accurate estimate of max heart rate. The next step is to use some percentages of this number to set up your zones. Setting five zones is usually done something like this:

Zone	% Max Heart Rate
1	50–59%
2	60–69%
3	70–79%
4	80–89%
5	90–100%

Voilà! You'd have your zones. But there's a problem. This method assumes that the zones will work the same for everyone. If two athletes, for example, both complete a workout at 90 percent of max the effort, the resulting physiological benefits will be the same. There's a great chance that they won't, however. To understand this dilemma, you must first come to grips with something called lactate threshold.

Lactate threshold (LT) is the level of intensity at which you begin to "redline." In other words, the effort above LT is so difficult that you find it difficult to continue. Your breathing is deep and forceful, you are about RPE 7, and you may experience a burning sensation in the working muscles. You can only maintain this level of effort for a few minutes up to an hour or so for a highly fit athlete. And the higher above LT the effort goes, the shorter the time it can be maintained.

The interesting thing about LT, and what makes using max heart rate an ineffective reference point for your zones, is that it can vary widely as a percent of max—anywhere from around 70 to 90 percent of max heart rate. Generally, the more fit the athlete, the higher the LT heart rate is as a percent of max.

So in our example above, even if the two athletes have exactly the same max heart rate, they could easily have different LTs as a percent of max. So if both trained at 85 percent of max and one has an LT at 80 percent of max heart rate she is working at a very hard effort—perhaps an RPE of 9. If the other athlete has an LT at 90 percent of max heart rate his RPE may be 6 when exercising at 85 percent of max. These are certainly not the same workout for these two individuals, nor are the physiological benefits going to be the same even though both athletes are exercising at the same 90 percent of max heart rate.

The lesson here, again, is not to use max heart rate as a reference point in setting up your heart rate zones. So what *should* you use, then?

Use LT. Since it is such a critical point in your effort range, it is the perfect reference point. The trick is finding out what your LT heart rate is. Let's find out how you can do that.

[Finding Your LT]

If LT is so important for determining your heart rate training zones, it's critical that you know yours and have some confidence that it is correct. How do you do that? The answer is testing. There are two broad categories—metabolic tests and field tests.

METABOLIC TESTING

At least once each year I have the athletes I coach tested at a facility that offers metabolic assessment. This is commonly referred to as a "VO_2max test." Most athletes think this test tells them what their potentials are for their sports. It does *not* tell you this, any more than a hard workout tells you potential. This test merely quantifies your current level of fitness and also pinpoints your LT heart rate.

Besides learning LT, from which I can set up heart rate zones for the athletes I coach, I also find such testing useful in discovering how fit the athletes are before planning the next few weeks of their training programs. Other information gleaned from the metabolic test includes bike power zones for cyclists and rowers, how much fat and carbohydrate are used at various intensities, and how efficiently the athletes move. Testing also helps to dial in each athlete's personal RPE on the 1 to 10 scale so that we can talk about effort more precisely in the future.

That's a lot of useful information for a coach, produced in a one-hour test. If you are self-coached, the technician can help you make

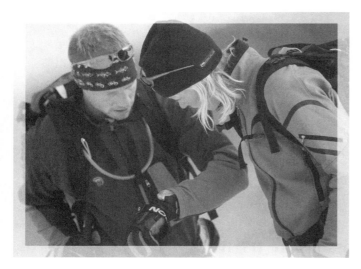

sense of the test results and may even offer suggestions on how to use the information to train more effectively. He or she can also help you determine your lactate threshold heart rate from the data and set up your zones accordingly. Be sure to tell the technician before the test that this is one of the main outcomes you want.

This test generally costs in the range of $100 to $200. Look for a facility that specializes in athlete testing, not one that caters to those at risk for heart disease or to aging populations. The latter will have different testing protocols and perspectives on the data. Although these are often referred to as "lab" tests, a recent trend is for physical therapy clinics, health clubs, bike shops, and running stores to offer such testing services.

By repeating the test at the start of each major period of the season, especially the Base 1, Build 1, and Peak periods (see Chapter 4 for details), you can closely monitor progress. Tests not only tell you how much progress you are making—and in a very precise way—but also serve as great motivators.

You can find testing centers throughout the United States that I recommend listed at www.TotalHRT.com.

FIELD TESTING

The beauty of the metabolic testing described above is precision. The technician who administers the test will attempt to control all the possible variables, such as temperature and humidity, standardization and calibration of equipment, warm-up, testing procedure, and more. By controlling such things the technician can be fairly confident that changes in results between tests are due to your fitness changing rather than to some external factors. The downside, of course, is cost. You pay for this precision. So you probably won't want to be tested this way too frequently. And yet, as mentioned, it's important that you check your LT heart rate and discover your current level of fitness fairly often—about every four to eight weeks is best. So what do you do?

The answer is field testing—tests you conduct on yourself in your normal training environment. This could be in a swimming pool, on a running track or velodrome, on a standard course you've selected, or indoors using available training equipment (for example, bicycle ergometer, rowing ergometer, or treadmill). While such testing is inexpensive, probably costing you nothing or at least very little per test, precision may be questionable.

Not only must you yourself control for such external variables as weather, equipment, warm-up, and procedure, you must also control your internal factors. What you eat and when you eat before testing can make a difference in the results. For example, a couple of cups of coffee before one test but not another may well produce two sets of heart rate numbers and throw off the results. Your emotional state can also have an impact on the test. If you are under a lot of stress before a test, heart rate will be affected. Time of day for the testing may even be a factor. And a critical variable is how well rested you are coming into the test. If the results are to be meaningful and give you guidance for future training, you must make the test conditions as precise as possible.

See "Common Field Tests for Lactate Threshold Heart Rate" (pages 44–45) for examples of ways to self-test. A purpose of each of these tests is to discover your lactate threshold heart rate. If done correctly, the results you get should be a good approximation of this and close to what would be discovered in a metabolic test. If the test is poorly conducted—meaning the variables described above are not controlled—the results may give you quite erroneous information. Basing your training on such data may be a waste of time and may even severely limit your growth as an athlete.

[When to Test]

Tests to determine LT are best done when you are rested, since fatigue, even slight, may well affect the results. And this is a good time to point out that LT also may vary from one day to the next, based on how well rested you are. On some days the effort you put out may seem harder, when compared with heart rate, than on other days. You're simply tired.

To make sure you're rested and ready for a test, make your training easy for three to five days before. Chapter 6 shows you how to do this by describing a periodized training program with several consecutive days for recovery built

in every three to four weeks. At the end of one of these R&R weeks is a good time to test.

[Confirming Test Results]

Regardless of the method you used to find your LT, you are now ready to set up your heart rate zones and start training with them. This is described in the next section. But once you've set up your zones it's a good idea to confirm your LT in the days and weeks following the test. It's possible that one or more uncontrolled variables affected the results or that the test was flawed in some way. For example, in a metabolic test this could result from the technician's not properly calibrating the test equipment. Or if you did a 30-minute field test you may have started out too fast and then faded near the end. This is common the first few times this test is done. Confirming your LT will ensure that your training is proceeding as intended.

Unfortunately, there is no objective, surefire way to confirm the test results. You'll base the decision largely on subjective comparisons. What you need to confirm is that the LT heart rate is about right—neither too high nor too low. Once you've repeated the LT-determination test a few times over the course of several weeks, you no longer need confirmation. By then you'll have it nailed down.

The easiest way to confirm the results of your test is to simply pay attention to your heart rate monitor while working out. On harder workouts, as heart rate rises and approaches your estimated LT, pay close attention to your breathing. It should become increasingly labored. At about your true LT the volume of air you are moving in and out should sharply rise. There is a fairly obvious change at this point that sports

Text continued on page 46.

COMMON FIELD TESTS FOR LACTATE THRESHOLD HEART RATE

The following are self-tests you can do to determine lactate threshold (LT) heart rate for your sport. Once you know LT heart rate, set up your heart rate training zones by finding your sport's heart rate table in Appendix 2. Find your LT heart rate in the bold numbers in the "5a" column. Reading the row both left and right of this number produces your heart rate zones.

30-MINUTE TEST

This is a simple test—but not easy. All you have to do is complete a 30-minute time trial on a constant course such as a flat road, slight uphill, or calm water. It may also be done indoors on an ergometer for your sport, such as a bike trainer, rower, or treadmill. Most athletes find this harder to do indoors than outdoors. If you decide to test indoors, be sure to have a fan or cool room to exercise in. Heat will adversely affect results. This test is best done alone, as having a partner may also affect the results.

Start by warming up adequately. You should have a sense of what that means for you, since it should be about the same as what you do before a race. Most athletes need at least 10 minutes of warm-up before this test. But you may want as much as 30 minutes.

Once warmed up and ready to go, immediately start the test. The key to this test is pacing. Almost everyone starts at too great an intensity and then fades in the last few minutes. It's not unusual to hear of athletes failing to finish the test the first time because of starting out too fast. Tell yourself you'll hold back just a little the first 10 minutes, and continually remind yourself of this once the test begins.

At exactly 10 minutes into the test click the lap button on your heart rate monitor. Then when the test ends, click the stop button. You now will have three heart rate-data points captured on your heart rate monitor—average heart rate for the first 10 minutes, average for the last 20 minutes, and average for the entire 30 minutes. The one we are interested in is your average for the last 20 minutes. This a good estimate of your LT heart rate. Use it to determine your heart rate zones, as described in this chapter.

Other good information to record from this test is your average velocity or power for the entire 30 minutes. For while your LT heart rate might not change much in subsequent tests, with improving fitness both velocity and power *will* change for the better.

GRADED EXERCISE TEST

This test is similar to what you would do in a test in a clinic or lab, but, of course, does not include the use of expensive metabolic assessment equipment. Besides a heart rate monitor, you will need an ergometer that's appropriate for your sport. This could be a treadmill for running, a stationary bike or indoor bicycle trainer, or a rowing ergometer. (This test does not work well for swimming unless you use a flume.) The ergometer must accurately display some output measure such as speed, pace, or watts. Be sure that the ergometer is set for the "manual" mode. You will also need an assistant to hold the heart rate monitor receiver (wristwatch) and record information.

The following is a description of how to conduct the test.

1. Warm up on the equipment for 10–15 minutes.

2. Set the machine to start the test at a very easy resistance—something that takes little effort to

do. Your RPE should be on the low end in the first minute—about 2 on the 1-to-10 scale.

3. Every minute increase the machine's resistance by a small amount. Your effort level will rise steadily. This continues until you are forced to stop because of fatigue.

4. Each minute, your assistant records the current level of output (speed, pace, power). At the end of each minute, tell your assistant how great your exertion is, using the 1-to-10 RPE scale described in this chapter (you might place the RPE page where it can be seen during the test).

5. Your assistant records your exertion rating and your heart rate at the end of the minute and assists you, if necessary, in changing the equipment to the next higher level of resistance.

4. The assistant also listens closely to your breathing to detect when it first becomes deep and forceful. This is the "VT," or ventilatory threshold, which correlates quite closely with lactate threshold. The more times your assistant helps you conduct this test, the better he or she will get at identifying the VT.

5. Continue the test by increasing the resistance every minute until you can no longer hold the output.

The following is an example of the data collected from such a test. The "Output" column is not specific to any particular sport or ergometer. Your numbers may well be different for each column, but this is generally the way it will look.

Output	Heart Rate	RPE
1.5	110	2
2.0	118	3
2.5	125	3
3.0	135	4
3.5	142	5
4.0	147	6
4.5	153	6
5.0	156	7 "VT"
5.5	159	7
6.0	163	8
6.5	165	9

Now that you have collected the data, it's time to locate your approximate lactate threshold (LT) heart rate. Use the following guidelines to do that.

1. If you really pushed yourself, your LT heart rate will be found in the last five data points. In the example above, the last five data points begin with an output of "4.5."

2. If an RPE of 7 is found in the last five data points, assume that where it first appears is your LT heart rate. If you did not push yourself to your limit on the test, assume that where you assigned a 7 RPE is your LT heart rate.

3. If RPE 7 occurs before the last five data points and your assistant's subjective identification of VT is found in that range, assume that this is your LT heart rate.

4. If neither RPE 7 nor your assistant's VT notation is found in the last five data points, then assume that your LT heart rate is the fifth one before the end of the test.

Applying these criteria to the example above, the LT heart rate is found to be 156 bpm. Realize that this is merely an estimate of your LT heart rate. You may get slightly different results with subsequent tests. But for now use this number to determine your heart rate zones, as described in this chapter.

scientists call the "ventilatory threshold" (VT). VT and LT heart rate occur almost simultaneously. Having paid close attention to breathing a few times in workouts, you'll be able to decide if your estimated LT is too high or too low. Make small adjustments to it and then train accordingly, as described in the next section.

Another subjective way to confirm your LT test result is to apply RPE, as described above, while you are working out. Since most people rate their exertion at about 7 on a 1-to-10 scale, when at LT you can again confirm your test results. When you realize you're working at a 7 RPE, take a glance at your heart rate monitor. You should see your tested LT. If not, make zone adjustments as necessary. But, again, realize that this is quite a subjective call. It's best not to make changes to your LT heart rate based on one such workout. Continue to monitor RPE and change your LT heart rate if it seems to be off the mark, based on several such subjective incongruities.

And finally, if you did a metabolic test to find LT, you could later do a field test to confirm results. Or use a different field test to confirm the results of your first field test.

THE HEART RATE ZONES

Once you have established your LT heart rate, it's time to set up your zones. To do this turn to Appendix 2. Here there are several tables for different sports. Find the table for your sport and then locate your LT heart rate in the bold listings under the "5a" column. Then by reading the row to the left and right of this number you will find all your heart rate target zones from

Zone 1 to Zone 5c. Each of these zones has a purpose and physiological benefit.

If you really examine all the tables closely, you'll notice that the percentages of LT are not the same for each zone across the spectrum of the sports. For example, for running Heart Rate Zone 2 is about 81 to 89 percent of LT, and for cycling Zone 2 is 85 to 90 percent of LT. The reason for this is that each of these sports has a unique metabolic response to exercise. The following is a brief description of each of the zones you'll find for your sport in Appendix 2.

[Zone 1: Active Recovery]

This is the lowest and easiest of the zones. Exercising in this zone will allow your body to recover from previous hard training. You can speed recovery in two ways. Zone 1 is referred to as "active recovery," meaning that the stresses are so low that the body should still be able to get back to a rested level. Even easier is "passive recovery," which essentially means resting without exercising at all. Highly fit and experienced athletes will find that Zone 1 promotes recovery. Inexperienced athletes and those who are at low levels of fitness should use passive rather than active recovery, especially following very challenging workouts.

[Zone 2: Aerobic Threshold]

Training in Zone 2 is the best way to improve your aerobic function without a huge requirement for recovery afterward. Chapter 4 explains how exercising in this zone, especially the upper half of it, builds aerobic threshold fitness—the basis for success in all endurance sports. Zone 2 is also sometimes called "extensive endurance," because a well-conditioned athlete can maintain this level of intensity for many hours.

Training in Zone 2 usually involves long, steady efforts in which you keep a close watch on your heart rate monitor. These steady workouts could be up to 4 hours, depending on your sport and level of fitness.

[Zone 3: Tempo]

This is sometimes referred to as the "gray zone" in some disciplines, because the physiological benefits are not much greater than those achieved in upper-Zone 2 training, although the need for recovery afterward is considerably greater. The next chapter will discuss this zone in greater detail.

Zone 3 workouts are either long, steady efforts or intervals, depending on fitness and your competitions. Races that are done in Zone 3 require a good deal of Zone 3 training and long, steady efforts. But if your competitions are raced well above or below Zone 3, then its value to you is limited.

[Zone 4: Sub-Lactate Threshold]

Zone 4 is the intensity that most athletes gravitate to in steady-state competitions lasting from a few minutes up to about 3 hours. At this level, acid production is significant but the body copes with it well. Going slightly above this zone—into Zone 5a—causes the production of so much acid that exercise duration is greatly limited. Zone 4 is highly effective for improving acid tolerance with long exercise bouts.

Training in Zone 4 usually involves long work intervals, such as 6 to 12 minutes, with recovery intervals that are only about one-fourth as long as the work intervals. So for 6-minute work intervals the recoveries would be about 90 seconds. These short recoveries keep acid levels high in the muscles to stimulate greater adaptation. A total of 20 to 60 minutes of total Zone 4 interval time within a single workout session is adequate to build fitness without severely prolonging recovery.

[Zone 5a: Lactate Threshold]

This is your LT intensity. You'll see in your sport's table in Appendix 2 that Zone 5a is quite small—only about 4 beats per minute. It's small because we want to use it to narrowly define your LT. At this level of intensity acid is beginning to accumulate in your muscles, in body fluids surrounding your muscles, and in your blood. Training here is very effective for developing endurance fitness.

Since even the most fit athletes can only maintain this intensity for an hour or so, interval training is very common for Zone 5a, and the procedure is the same as that used in Zone 4.

[Zone 5b: Aerobic Capacity]

At Zone 5b you are exercising well above LT. At the upper end of this zone you are at your aerobic capacity—the highest level of intensity at which your aerobic system is fully functioning. In fact, at this upper limit you can probably only maintain the effort for a few minutes. Zone 5b training is the most effective heart rate zone for improving aerobic capacity, since it maximally stresses the aerobic system, but such workouts incur a great recovery cost. This sort of training should be done infrequently, if at all, for most endurance sports. All Zone 5b training is done

HR ZONE	RPE ZONE	TITLE	PURPOSE	TYPICAL DURATION
1	1–2	Active Recovery	Actively recover from previous hard training	Limited only by sleep
2	3–4	Aerobic Threshold	Build aerobic endurance	<12 hours
3	5	Tempo	Challenge aerobic system	<8 hours
4	6–7	Sub-Lactate Threshold	Improve acid tolerance for long endurance	<3 hours
5a	8	Lactate threshold	Build LT performance	<1 hour
5b	9	Aerobic Capacity	Maximally challenge aerobic system	<20 minutes
5c	10	Anaerobic Capacity	Maximally challenge anaerobic system	<2 minutes

Table 3.2. Heart Rate and RPE Zones

as intervals, generally with equally long work and recovery intervals. The intervals should be 2 to 6 minutes' duration, depending on which end of Zone 5b you are exercising in. An example of such a workout is 3-minute intervals with 3-minute recoveries. Generally, 15 minutes of Zone 5b work intervals within a single session is adequate to produce results without seriously overtaxing your recovery.

[Zone 5c: Anaerobic Capacity]

This is the extreme upper end of your heart rate training zones and where your max heart rate may be found. Training at such an intensity is not recommended for most endurance sports. An exception is events in which the outcome is often decided by a sprint that lasts only a few seconds, as in road cycling. In fact, since you can only maintain such an effort for a few seconds up to perhaps a minute, heart rate is not gener-

ally effective for gauging it. It takes from several seconds to a few minutes for heart rate to climb to such a level, so heart rate may not attain this rate until after the high effort is complete. Athletes who must train their anaerobic capacity are advised to rely on RPE, velocity, or power.

Table 3.2 summarizes the details of these heart rate zones and compares them with RPE.

THE HEART OF THE MATTER

Having read this chapter, you should now understand how to set your heart rate training zones using your lactate threshold (LT) as a reference point. Once this is done, your heart rate monitor becomes more than just a novelty; it becomes a tool that can help take your athletic performance to a higher level as a result of better training. The next chapter shows you how to do that.

4

BEYOND THE BASICS

If you've been using your monitor to train as most athletes use it, you've probably done little more than observe your heart rate while exercising and then record your average heart rates in your training diary following workouts. That's a good starting place for using your device and is basic to monitoring your progression. But it is not very enlightening or helpful when it comes to knowing how to train effectively. The purpose of this chapter is to take you beyond simply using the instantaneous and average heart rate features by giving you more advanced tools to help you achieve your performance goals. Along the way you'll learn more about your body and how a heart rate monitor can make you a more fit athlete.

THE AEROBIC THRESHOLD

Chapter 3 described the lactate threshold as the key reference point in setting your heart rate training zones. Let's review, because this is a critical point, not only in setting your heart rate zones but also in understanding and improving your training and racing. Here is how the previous chapter explained it:

Lactate threshold (LT) is the level of intensity at which you begin to "red-line." In other words, the effort above LT is so difficult that you find it difficult to continue. Your breathing is deep and forceful, you are about RPE 7, and you may experience a burning sensation in the working muscles. You can only maintain this level of effort for a few minutes, or up to an hour or so for a highly fit athlete. And the higher above LT the effort goes, the shorter the time it can be maintained.

Knowing your LT heart rate will allow you to train precisely at those times when you're in the upper zones, which is critical to success in endurance sports. It is known, for example, that training right at or slightly below your LT heart rate boosts LT fitness without the need for the very long recovery that necessarily follows training above the LT. Highly intense workouts above the LT, while sometimes necessary, depending on your sport, demand a lengthy recovery during the following days, costing you valuable training time. So staying just below LT helps to produce excellent fitness without a lot of downtime. This knowledge of where your LT heart rate occurs is also valuable information for races, especially those that last longer than one hour. For such events, knowing LT heart rate will allow you to correctly pace yourself to produce a good performance without undue fatigue.

By now you should have the basic idea of how to find and use LT heart rate in training and racing. So let's introduce another handy reference point—the *aerobic threshold*. I use the abbreviation "AeT" when referring to aerobic threshold so as not to confuse it with another abbreviation you may have seen used in magazines and books—"AT," as shorthand for *anaerobic threshold*. I won't concern you with the details of this term. It is essentially just another way of saying "lactate threshold." So the moniker AeT makes sure you don't get your thresholds mixed up. To help with that I won't bring up AT again.

AeT is a lower level of intensity than LT but also important to your training. Training at this intensity is used to fully develop your aerobic system fitness, just as LT training is used to create high-intensity fitness. Aerobic fitness is critical to success in endurance events. When it is well developed, your cardiorespiratory system (heart, lungs, and blood) is capable of delivering large quantities of oxygen to the working muscles, which gladly accept and use it to produce energy from body fat to keep you moving.

Recall that LT was defined as the point at which lactate and acidic hydrogen ions begin to accumulate in your blood as you steadily increase the intensity of a workout. Long before you got to this LT heart rate point, as the workout was getting harder, you would have passed through AeT heart rate. At AeT several physiological changes can be identified that help mark when it occurs. For example, if we could measure how much air you breathe in and out in 1 minute during a workout, we'd find a point where it suddenly increases beyond the light breathing of easy exercise. This is your AeT. At this same intensity point, the amount of carbon dioxide you breathe out would also increase suddenly.

With sophisticated testing equipment we could identify your heart rate at this intensity by measuring these variables. There's another way I've found that is a lot easier—and cheaper. For most endurance athletes, AeT occurs at about the lower end of heart rate Zone 2. That's why it's called the Aerobic Threshold Zone. At the

start of Zone 2 your RPE is about 3 on the 10-point scale described in Chapter 3. By the upper end of Zone 2, your RPE is about 4 and is marked by some difficulty in talking with your training partner.

So why is AeT important to training and fitness? Besides the changes in your ventilation rate and carbon dioxide production, other changes are happening as you arrive at AeT intensity in a workout. One of the most important of these changes has to do with your muscles. Let's learn a little more about muscle physiology to better understand this important point.

Basically, you have two types of fibers that make up your muscles—slow twitch and fast twitch. Slow twitch, also called "Type I," are the muscles that make us good at endurance sports, such as marathon running, triathlon, rowing, bicycle road racing, and mountain biking. These muscles rely on oxygen and fat to produce energy. But while they have good endurance properties and can contract repeatedly for long durations, they are not strong when compared with fast twitch fibers.

Fast twitch fibers, or "Type II," are found in abundance in elite power athletes in sports such as sprinting, shot put, football, and tennis. These muscles produce great power compared with slow twitch but have poor endurance qualities. They fatigue easily. Type II muscles do not require as much oxygen to produce energy, and they rely mostly on carbohydrate for fuel.

So it's easy to see that as an endurance athlete you'd prefer to have a lot of slow twitch muscles. Unfortunately, it appears that muscle type is largely determined by genetics. If you don't have much in the way of slow twitch muscles, have a serious talk with your parents.

But there's hope if you are a natural-born power athlete aspiring to do endurance events. Fast twitch muscles actually are found in two varieties in everyone—Type IIa and Type IIb. Type IIb is the pure power muscle. Type IIa, however, has some slow twitch characteristics, and, better yet, is highly trainable. If you do a lot of endurance training, Type IIa's endurance qualities will improve while they lose some of their power ability. That's just one more of the human body's beautiful features.

There's one more thing about muscle you need to know to fully appreciate Zone 2–AeT training. The nervous system has a preferential way of selecting muscles when it's necessary to do some work. At the easiest level, as when exercising very slowly, say at RPE 1 or 2, or when lifting a light weight, your body calls on the Type I muscles first. So Type IIa and Type IIb don't do much of anything and are basically resting. But if you step up the intensity just a bit, the nervous system eventually needs more than just Type I to do the job, so it next calls on Type IIa muscle fibers. If you decide to go even faster or lift an even heavier load, more and more muscle is called on, with Type IIb being recruited last. When you are sprinting all out or trying to set a personal best record in weight lifting, you are using all three muscle types.

The most important lesson here is that Type IIa fibers are recruited at about your AeT heart rate—or approximately at the low end of Zone 2. That makes exercising in Zone 2 an extremely effective use of your training time. Zone 1 is not as effective at developing the aerobic potential of Type IIa muscle, and Zone 3, while it will enhance Type IIa endurance characteristics, is more physically demanding and so has a longer recovery period, in the following hours

and days, than Zone 2 workouts. Chapter 5 describes the details of Zone 2 workouts.

The bottom line is that Zone 2 should be emphasized in your training to make you a more complete endurance athlete. Regardless of your sport, a sizable amount of your endurance training should be at and just above AeT heart rate. This raises the issue of how much training you should do in each heart rate zone.

TIME BY TRAINING ZONE

How much time should you spend in each heart rate zone over the entire season? This is a question asked by many athletes and with good reason. Knowing the answer will lead to purposeful and effective training. Unfortunately, it's not an easy one to answer.

Training intensity for a given workout is chosen for several reasons, perhaps the most important of which is the event for which you're training. There are tremendous differences between preparing for a triathlon and a bicycle road race, even though the durations of these two events and the average heart rates they produce may be exactly the same. A bicycle race is often determined by who has the most power in a sprint toward the finish line lasting only a few seconds, even though the race may last several grueling hours. But in triathlon a sprint seldom determines the outcome. The bike race also has widely varying intensities, from very easy to very hard, occurring frequently throughout. The triathlon, by contrast, is a steady effort from start to finish. Obviously, one cannot train with the same intensities and in the same way for both events.

Let's get back to the original question: How much time should you spend in each heart rate zone over the course of a season? It's apparent from the example that there is no single answer that can satisfy the needs of every athlete in every sport, since intensity and duration of events vary considerably. But we may be able to make some broad generalizations by race duration and race type. Figures 4.1 to 4.5 provide a rough approximation of what the time distributions might look like. These should be viewed as general guidelines only, not as chiseled-in-stone standards to be achieved.

Realize that if we look at all the heart rate data for a given athlete for an entire season, there will always be a lot of time spent in Zone 1. That zone is also highly represented because of the nature of training, with recovery days, workout warm-ups and cool-downs, and low-intensity recoveries during interval workouts.

Let's also view the resulting distributions by event duration, using 3 and 8 hours as standards, and by event nature—steady-state pacing (as in a marathon) or variably paced (as in a bicycle road race).

Notice that there aren't any numbers or percentages on these figures. That's because there are simply too many variables to nail it down that tightly. Instead, these variables have to do with the nature and duration of the event—training for a 4-hour hilly race is different than training for a 7-hour flat race—and with individual differences. Some people simply need more anaerobic training than others. There is no right amount of zone time for everyone—even for athletes doing the same event. The figures are merely meant to generally show how time by heart rate zones should be distributed, not to give you the ultimate answer.

If we created such a graph for most self-coached athletes, we would probably find

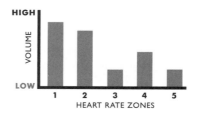

Fig. 4.1. Volume of Training by Heart Rate Zones Steady-State Events Less Than About 3 Hours

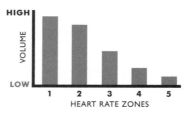

Fig. 4.2. Volume of Training by Heart Rate Zones Steady-State Events Less Than About 8 Hours

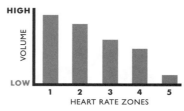

Fig. 4.3. Volume of Training by Heart Rate Zones Steady-State Events of About 3–8 Hours

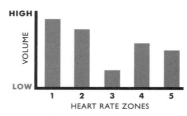

Fig. 4.4. Volume of Training by Heart Rate Zones Variably Paced Events Less Than About 3 Hours

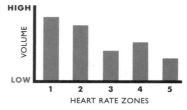

Fig. 4.5. Volume of Training by Heart Rate Zones Variably Paced Events Longer Than About 3 Hours

something considerably different than what is suggested in these figures. Regardless of the nature and duration of the event, there would be a peak in Zone 3, with less time in both the lower and higher zones. The reason for this is that most athletes training without a planned purpose gravitate to the middle by making their easy days too hard and, as a result of the fatigue from the "easy" days, making their hard days too easy. So the middle ground—Zone 3—is dominant.

The take-home lesson here is that training intensity should reflect not only the demands of building solid, basic fitness, but also the intensity of the events for which you train. Because every endurance event is unique and places specific demands on certain zones, your training must emphasize those same zones so that you can become fully fit and ready to compete.

PULSE, PACE, AND POWER

As mentioned earlier, observing the instantaneous heart rate reading on your monitor while working out does not tell you anything unless you compare the number to some known reference point, such as LT heart rate or AeT heart rate. Or, of course, you can simply compare the number you are seeing to your heart rate zones and know what it means. Another option is to compare your heart rate with non-heart-rate measures of intensity. For example, Chapter 3 described how you could confirm your zones by comparing heart rate with RPE (Rating of Perceived Exertion) using a 1-to-10-point scale with 1 representing extremely easy and 10 extremely hard. At the moment during a workout when you rate exertion as 8, your heart rate should be quite close to LT. And as described earlier in this chapter, when RPE is about 3 or 4 you are close to AeT heart rate.

While this works for most athletes, some have trouble getting RPE dialed in. After all, it is entirely subjective. There is a learning curve associated with effectively using RPE. The best way to become accurate with RPE is to use it frequently. Several times during every workout, take mental note of how you rate the exertion level. Don't look for right or wrong ratings; simply trust your intuition. It will take time to establish consistency.

RPE, however, will always be somewhat questionable, since it is subjective. That will be especially evident when you train with other athletes. What feels like a 7 when you are alone may get rated as a 5 when you have a training partner. Motivation and inward concentration, both of which are affected when you're around other athletes, play a big role in judging RPE levels.

What would be even better than RPE is to compare heart rate with objective measures of intensity, especially "output" measures. As explained earlier, heart rate is an "input" indicator of intensity. It tells you how hard you are working—not how much work is being accomplished. The bottom line in sports is what you are accomplishing—not how hard you are trying. For example, at the end of a running race the officials do not award prizes to those with the highest heart rates (input); the prizes go to those who ran the fastest (output). In fact, the winner of the race could have been working less hard than the person who finished last. This doesn't make heart rate less important in judging intensity. Knowing your input is still a critical factor in performance. So is output. Comparing them is especially effective.

Comparing heart rate input with some sort of output measure is particularly helpful when you want to know how your fitness is progressing. While heart rate will change little over the course of the season, once you are in decent condition, output should change considerably at any given heart rate. Let's go back to our running example to understand this.

At the start of the race season in March an athlete runs a 10k road race in 40 minutes at an average heart rate of 160. In September on the same course she runs 38 minutes at an average heart rate of 160. What have we learned about this runner? We simply know that her fitness has improved in six months, because she's running faster at the same heart rate. We could even quantify her fitness and say it had improved by 5 percent (2-minute improvement divided by 40 minutes).

Comparing heart rate with output measures makes your monitor an even more valuable training tool than simply comparing heart rates with zones.

[Heart Rate and Pace]

As shown in this example, comparing heart rate with pace is a great way to know how your training is going and whether your fitness is improving. Many sports rely on pace to gauge performance—running, swimming, and cross-country skiing are a few common examples. In these sports comparing heart rate to pace is an effective way of gauging progress.

The problem with pace is that you don't always have a measured course with frequent distance markers that can be used to compute how fast you are going. Another is that it requires some mental gymnastics while exercising. That can be prove difficult, especially when fatigue is setting in late in a hard workout. But, fortunately, recent technological developments

make it possible to have real-time pace data displayed on your wrist along with heart rate. With a Global Positioning Satellite (GPS) device or accelerometer, pacing information is at your fingertips. This allows you to compare heart rate and pace instantaneously and to critically analyze them after the workout or race by downloading the data to your computer.

As with all such high-tech gear, these devices can be expensive. GPS units start at about $150 for pacing information only, which requires wearing a separate heart rate monitor. A GPS device with a heart rate function built in costs about $350. Accelerometers, which also include a heart rate display, such as the Polar S725x and the RS200sd, start at about $220.

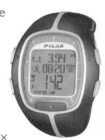

RS200sd

Heart rate may be compared with pace during any steady-state workout segment that lasts more than about 5 minutes. A shorter segment may be used for comparison if you are diligent about bringing heart rate up to a standard level before beginning the segment to be analyzed. Two of the best workouts to do such comparisons with are AeT and LT workouts. Since these are such critical stages in the training process (see Chapter 7) and workouts that should be done frequently, comparing pace and heart rate at these times can provide good insights into your progress. It is best to do such steady-paced workouts on a flat course or running track.

These workouts are described in detail in Chapter 5, but they are quite simple, involving long, steady efforts at AeT and LT heart rate ranges. Then after the workout is done you download the pacing-heart rate device's data to your computer and analyze it in a graphic display. Figure 4.6 illustrates what you would want to see

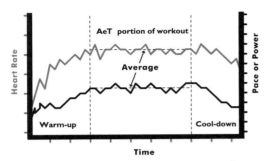

Fig. 4.6. Heart rate compared with pace or power during an AeT workout. Note the parallel (coupled) nature of the heart rate and pace (or power) lines during the AeT portion indicating good aerobic fitness.

in the computer display of a steady AeT workout. Note that following the warm-up the athlete holds a fairly steady AeT heart rate for several minutes and the average pacing line parallels the average heart rate line. Heart rate and pace remain "coupled" for the entire AeT portion of the workout. This coupling indicates that for this duration the athlete is in good aerobic condition.

Figure 4.7 reveals that the athlete is *not* in good aerobic condition beyond about the halfway point of the steady AeT segment, since pace begins to drop off even though heart rate remains steady. Heart rate and pace are "decoupling" at roughly the halfway mark. The athlete's aerobic fitness on that day was good only for the duration of the coupled portion. Essentially, what we are measuring here is cardiac drift, which was described in Chapter 2. Even though it is apparent that heart rate is not rising in the AeT segment of the workout, the fact that pace is falling confirms the drift. If the athlete were maintaining a steady pace instead of a steady heart rate—another option when doing this workout—heart rate would have drifted upward.

It is even possible to precisely measure how much decoupling is taking place in such a work-

out by comparing pace with heart rate for each half of the AeT segment. Here's how to calculate the rate of decoupling:

STEP 1. Determine average pace and average heart rate for each half of the AeT (or LT) portion of the workout.

STEP 2. Divide the average pace for each half by the average heart rate for each half.

STEP 3. Subtract the second-half quotient from the first-half quotient. If the remainder is a negative number, which will usually be the case if the steady-state portion is long enough, you know you slowed down in the second half.

STEP 4. Divide the remainder by the first half quotient. This is a percentage that tells you how much drift (decoupling) was experienced during the workout.

That's a lot of math. Let's use an example to make it easier to follow.

A runner does a 30-minute AeT-segment workout. In the first half he averages 7 minutes and 30 seconds per mile (7.5/mile) and an average heart rate of 132 beats per minute (bpm). In the second half he has an average pace of 8

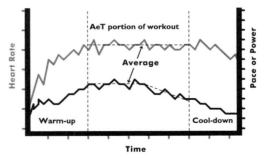

Fig. 4.7. Heart rate compared with pace or power during an AeT workout. Note the decoupling of the pace (or power) line from the heart rate line during the latter half of the AeT portion. This indicates poor aerobic fitness.

minutes per mile (8.0/mile) at the same 132 bpm. Here's how the steps from above would be applied to this situation:

STEP 1. First half average pace was 7.5 and heart rate was 132. Second half average pace was 8.0 and heart rate was 132.

STEP 2. First half: 7.5 ÷ 132 = 0.0568. Second half: 8.0 ÷ 132 = 0.0606.

STEP 3. 0.0568 − 0.0606 = −0.0038 (a negative number, indicating decoupling).

STEP 4. −0.0038 ÷ 0.0568 = −.066 (6.6% decoupling).

When an athlete is in good aerobic condition, decoupling should be less than 5 percent. Athletes who are in excellent physical condition decouple less than 1 percent, even for the longest AeT-portion workouts.

As mentioned, Chapter 5 will discuss both AeT- and LT-segment workouts in greater detail and provide suggested durations to use for the steady-state segments by sport.

[Heart Rate and Power]

Pace or speed is not an effective output measure for cycling because of the much greater effect of wind at the higher velocities of the sport. Power, expressed in wattage, is a better metric to track output intensity for cycling. In fact, given a choice for any sport, power measurement would be preferable to pace since power is unaffected by uphills, downhills, headwinds, and tailwinds. Pace varies considerably under such conditions. Power measurement, however, is only available in a few sports now.

Cycling was the first sport to use powermeters to gauge intensity. These devices are built

into the bike at the rear hub, bottom bracket, or crankset. Powermeters are pretty pricey, starting at about $1,200 as of this writing. As with most new technology, the prices will probably come down in a few years as competition increases and as meters' popularity grows.

Less-expensive options are available to estimate the cyclist's power. One such device is the Polar Power System combined with the Polar S720i or Polar S725x heart rate monitors. Instead of measuring power using strain gauges as most powermeters do, the Polar device measures both chain tension, using a sensor on the chain stay, and chain speed, using a sensor on the rear pulley. From these measurements it calculates power. The advantage of such a system is reduced weight—a major factor when climbing hills on a bike. The Polar Power System costs about $350.

Polar Power Sensor.

For the triathlete or cross trainer, the Polar S725X is a good option since it may be used both as an accelerometer to measure pace while running and as a power device for cycling.

Power measurement devices may also be found in ergometers used for indoor training for cycling and rowing, and even on some treadmills. Someday you may even see power devices built into running shoes with a transmitted display to your wrist, although the cost of the technology will have to come down considerably for this to happen.

Following a bike workout you can download a powermeter and compare wattage with heart rate in much the same way it is done with pace. The resulting graphs will look much like those

TEMPO TIME TRIAL

COURSE SELECTION

Choose a Tempo Time Trial (TTT) course you can continue to use throughout the season. The best course is flat, has no or very little traffic, has no stop streets, and is out-and-back or circular to reduce the effect of wind. For a runner this might be a track, a cyclist could use a velodrome or isolated road, and a cross-country skier could find a protected and groomed track. The course should take about 6 to 12 minutes to complete at Zone 3.

You may also use an indoor ergometer for your sport (treadmill, rower, stationary bike), but be aware that poor calibration or heavy use of the equipment in a public facility may affect the results of your test.

SCHEDULING

Do a TTT every three to four weeks throughout the season to measure changes in fitness. This is best done after several days of recovery near the end of an R&R week (see Chapter 6 for details on R&R weeks).

TEST HEART RATE

To determine the upper end of the TTT heart rate range used in the test, subtract 9 from your LT heart rate. To establish the lower end of the range, subtract 11 from your LT heart rate. This 3-beats-per-minute range is the standard heart rate target range you will use for all future TTT tests, even if your LT heart rate changes a bit.

PREPARATION

It's important to control as many variables as possible when doing a TTT. For best results do it at about the same time of day for each test. Eat and drink in much the same way before each TTT. Use the same equipment configured in the same way.

Warm-Up

Gradually warm up on your test course for 10 to 20 minutes, allowing heart rate to rise steadily. In the last 5 minutes of the warm-up slowly elevate your heart rate to the lower end of the test range (11 beats per minute below LT heart rate). As soon as the test-range heart rate is achieved, click the lap button on your heart rate monitor and start the test.

THE TEST

Watch your heart rate closely throughout the test, being careful to stay in the 3-beat range. Speed up or slow down in small increments to control heart rate. During the test do not concern yourself with time—only heart rate. As you cross the finish line on your course, again click the lap button to capture your course time and average heart rate. Start a short and easy cool-down.

TEST DATA

Record your time for the course in your training diary, along with average heart rate. Compare the time with previous results of this same test. If you have done a good job of controlling the variables (weather, equipment, nutrition, warm-up), the time differences will reflect how your fitness is changing.

shown in Figures 4.6 and 4.7. And the heart rate–vs.–power data may be analyzed in exactly the same way as described in the above "Heart Rate and Pace" section. What you are looking for is the heart rate and power averages for a steady-state workout portion to remain coupled, with less than 5 percent drift. How long you should be able to maintain this coupling with minimal drift is explained in Chapter 5. Of course, there are many other ways to use a powermeter in training, which are also described in Chapter 5.

HOW ARE YOU DOING?

This chapter has thrown a lot of advanced heart rate training concepts at you. While there is no doubt that applying what is described here will help you grow as an athlete, it does take time to gather and analyze the data. Athletes who enjoy precisely measuring and evaluating their fitness are some mix of scientist, engineer, and accountant. Not everyone is into measuring the smallest details of their workouts. It's quite possible that you simply do not want to download your workout, graph the results, and calculate the smallest details of your fitness, even if it promises to make you a better athlete. So let's step back and look at some simpler ways of using your heart rate monitor to measure performance.

One of the most basic uses of a heart rate monitor—one that every athlete should include in training—is measuring the progress of aerobic fitness. You can do two simple self-tests to find out how your training is going. They work on the same principle as the other analysis methods in this chapter but aren't nearly as complex. The principle behind each of these methods may be expressed in either of two ways:

As aerobic fitness improves, heart rate decreases at a standard output.

or

As aerobic fitness improves, output increases at a standard heart rate.

The AeT workout discussed earlier in this chapter and illustrated in Figure 4.6 is a good example of this principle in action. The athlete holds a standard heart rate during a workout and observes pace or power to see what it does. This workout could be done weekly (and should be done at certain times in the season) and the progression of output compared over time. If you are becoming more aerobically fit, your pace or power will improve at a given heart rate. Every few weeks you will see small changes, with pace getting faster or power increasing.

Let's look at an example of how an AeT workout can also be a test. Every week for four weeks a runner runs on a standard course and maintains an average AeT heart rate of 132 for an hour. Each time average pace is determined for the workout. In week 1 the average pace was 8 minutes per mile. By week 4 the pace is 7 minutes 30 seconds per mile. The runner's aerobic fitness has definitely improved since the pace is faster even though heart rate has not changed. So this series of workouts that was done with the intent of improving fitness also doubles as a test, indicating the progress of the runner's fitness.

The problem with determining progress this way is that our runner may not want to do a 1-hour AeT run weekly throughout the season, and does not need to. As Chapter 7 explains, there needs to be variety in your training, not only for mental well-being but also to stimulate the development of all aspects of fitness. The AeT run is also too long, requiring too great a cost in the form of recovery afterward. It would be preferable to have a much shorter test that also precisely measures aerobic fitness changes over time. Here are two such tests.

[Tempo Time Trial]

This is a test that takes only a few minutes and can be done every three to four weeks to get a good idea of how your fitness is progressing. It's called a "Tempo" Time Trial because it is conducted in heart rate Zone 3, which puts you at tempo pace or tempo power. Zone 3 is a good intensity for such testing, since it is hard enough to make you work but not so hard as to require a long recovery period if the test is short enough. The best time to do this test is near the end of a rest and recovery week (see Chapters 6 and 7 for details on R&R weeks).

The "Tempo Time Trial" sidebar on page 58 provides the details of how to do such a time

RAMP TEST

COURSE SELECTION

The Ramp test should be done on a well-maintained and calibrated ergometer appropriate for your sport. This is critical to the results. If the equipment varies from one test to the next, you won't know whether the changes measured are due to your fitness or to the ergometer's resistance.

SCHEDULING

As with the TTT, the Ramp test should be done every three to four weeks throughout the season. Do the test after several days of recovery near the end of an R&R week (see Chapter 6 for details on R&R weeks).

TEST OUTPUT

The Ramp test is conducted in five stages, with the first four lasting 3 minutes each and the fifth being a 1-minute recovery stage. The first stage is done at a low output (pace, speed, or power). Each subsequent stage increases the workload in measured and consistent increments, forcing you to work harder. The fourth stage should end with heart rate being just under your LT heart rate. So you may need to experiment the first time you do this test to get the stage workloads right. Here are examples of stages, with output being measured in power (watts), velocity (miles per hour), and pace (minutes per mile).

STAGE	WATTS	MILES/HOUR	MINUTES/MILE
1 (3 min.)	110	12	8.5
2 (3 min.)	140	15	8.0
3 (3 min.)	170	18	7.5
4 (3 min.)	200	21	7.0
5 (1 min.)	0	0	0

PREPARATION

For best results the Ramp test should be done at about the same time of day each time. Eat and drink the same way before each test. Use the

trial for sports like running, cycling, rowing, and cross-country skiing.

[Ramp Test]

While the TTT kept your heart rate the same and measured the output (time), the Ramp test is based on a fixed output and measures heart rate as the variable to determine changes in fitness. This test is best done on an ergometer such as an indoor bicycle trainer, rowing machine, or treadmill. For best results the ergometer should be calibrated so that you know it provides a consistent workload from one test to the next. If you can't be sure of the reliability of the equipment, it is best to do the TTT to measure your fitness instead.

The "Ramp Test" sidebar below describes this test.

[How Are You Doing?]

The purpose of these tests is to measure changes in aerobic fitness throughout the sea-

same equipment, configured in the same way. Use the same stage progressions each time you do this test.

Warm-Up

Gradually warm up on the ergometer for 10 to 20 minutes, allowing heart rate to rise steadily as you increase the workload.

THE TEST

When you are ready to start the test, go to the predetermined Stage 1 output level (see Test Output on page 60), and click the lap button on your heart rate monitor. Hold this output for 3 minutes. At the end of 3 minutes, click the lap button again to capture your heart rate at that time and immediately increase the workload to Stage 2 output level. Continue in this same way through Stage 4. At the end of Stage 4, when you click the lap button, stop and remain standing or sitting without moving for 1 minute. At the end of that minute, click the lap button for the last time. Then begin an easy cool-down.

TEST DATA

You will have captured five important data points on your heart rate monitor. On some devices this will be the instantaneous heart rate at the end of 1 minute. On others it will be the average heart rate for the completed stage. Add these five heart rate numbers and you have a total, called your Ramp Score. Record this number in your training diary for future reference and comparison. Here is an example of the collected data for a bicycle rider with a LT heart rate of 150:

STAGE	WATTS	HEART RATE
1	110	99
2	140	112
3	170	131
4	200	145
5	Stop	88
Ramp Score	–	575

Over the course of a few weeks your Ramp Score will decrease as your aerobic fitness improves. An increase in Ramp Score indicates a loss of aerobic fitness.

son. If everything went as planned with your training and the tests were conducted flawlessly, you should see small, positive fitness changes every three to four weeks. But since these changes are so tiny (generally on the order of less than 1 percent), and since the potential variables (especially weather and equipment calibration) are so great, it's quite possible that you'll see more of a "ratcheting up" of fitness. One test may show a slight increase in fitness and the next, just four weeks later, a decrease. There may even be small, unexplainable shifts in the short term simply because we are humans and not robots. We have good days and bad. These things just happen. Expect them and don't be disappointed when they occur.

Over the course of several testing sessions, however, you should see improvement if your training was purposeful and consistent. By using the same test and then recording the results each time in a training diary, you'll be able to track changes from month to month and season to season. This allows you to compare training methods and learn what works—or doesn't work—for you.

THE **HEART** OF THE MATTER

In this chapter you learned about the aerobic threshold (AeT), how important it is for fitness, and how to improve and even measure it with your heart rate monitor. For most fit athletes, the AeT occurs at about the low end of heart rate Zone 2. Training at or just above this heart rate produces positive physiological changes, such as causing the Type IIa muscle fibers to take on more of the characteristics of Type I (slow twitch) muscle fibers. This benefits endurance.

By measuring cardiac drift, using the concept of the decoupling of heart rate with either pace or power, it is possible to know when basic aerobic fitness is fully achieved.

This chapter also explored how much time you should spend in each training zone over a season. You learned that it is not possible to offer a formula that works for every athlete in every sport. There are simply too many variables. But general suggestions were offered on what that time distribution should look like by broad sport categories.

Comparing heart rate with an output measure such as pace or power was also shown to be an effective way of gauging overall progress, since output measures vary greatly throughout the season even though heart rate may experience only slight changes. The Tempo Time Trial and the Ramp test were suggested as tools to measure these changes and gauge fitness improvement.

In the next chapter you'll learn how to use the heart rate zones described in Chapter 3 in your training and racing.

5

USING

YOUR ZONES

By now you should have a good understanding of your heart, your heart rate monitor, how to set up your training zones, and some advanced concepts used in heart rate training. Knowing all this will make you a better athlete. In this chapter we'll get down to the nitty-gritty—how to actually use your heart rate zones in workouts. But before doing that, let's get a handle on a central concept of heart rate–based workouts.

You can use a heart rate monitor in training in two ways—*prescriptively* and *postscriptively*. The most commonly used method is prescriptive, meaning that you plan the workout based on targeted heart rate zones and then observe heart rate throughout the workout to make sure you are achieving the intended intensities. After the workout, if you like, you can download the data file to a computer and analyze the results, as described in Chapter 4. Postscriptive use, by contrast, means doing the workout based on feel, your own rating of perceived exertion (RPE) as described in Chapter 3, or some other measure of intensity such as pace or power, but without watching heart rate during the workout. Then, afterward, you download the file and see how you did, heart-rate-wise.

This chapter will teach you how to use a heart rate monitor prescriptively.

Along the way we'll take a look at how to design heart rate–based workouts and how to race using heart rate as an intensity governor. After reading this chapter you will be able to design a workout that includes warm-up, one or more mainsets, and cool-down, and will understand how to select a heart rate zone to set the upper limit on how much you push yourself in a race.

WORKOUTS AND ZONES

Should I warm up before a workout? How much? How hard? Do I need a cool-down at the end? How long? How easy? What types of workouts can I do to build fitness? Let's answer these fundamental heart rate training questions before moving on to the heart of the matter—workouts for each zone.

[Warm-Up and Cool-Down]

Warming up before a workout has a long but checkered history in the scientific research. Some studies have shown it to be beneficial, while others have found no or very little benefit. Most athletes, coaches, and exercise physiologists, however, believe in and use warm-up to prepare for the more intense activity to follow. Part of the benefit is undoubtedly related to the psychology of sport—warming up is assumed to be beneficial, so the athlete feels better prepared by it.

Those studies that have found a benefit indicate that it may help prevent injury while refining skills and improving coordination. These studies have shown that the warmed-up muscle temperature is higher, muscle acidity is less, and oxygen uptake is greater—all good things—after a warm-up when compared with no warm-up. For normally sedentary people who decide to exercise, warming up may be even more critical, as sudden exertion can trigger what the medical community calls *myocardial infarction,* or heart attack.

There are two types of warm-up: general and specific. General warm-up involves the use of stretching, calisthenics, and body movement for "loosening up" before starting an endurance workout or competition. This is probably less effective than specific warm-up involving low-intensity activity in your sport. For example, a runner would be better advised to run slowly to warm up for a running race rather than doing calisthenics. This is not to say that general warm-up is totally ineffective. There may well be times when specific warm-up is not possible, as when mountain bikers are corralled for 10 or more minutes before the start of their race. At such times stretching and general body movement may be marginally more effective than doing nothing.

The duration and intensity of the ensuing exercise also play a role in warming up. The shorter and more intense the race or workout, the longer the warm-up should be. The opposite also holds true: The longer and less intense the workout or race, the shorter the warm-up. Workouts done in heart rate Zone 1, for example, require no warm-up at all, but a Zone 5b interval workout is best preceded by a long,

thorough warm-up. Some long races may require a long warm-up if they are expected to start fast. This is often the case, for example, in multihour, bicycle road races for the lower participant categories. A short warm-up may take only 10 minutes, while a long one could last 45 minutes to an hour for a highly fit athlete doing a very short race.

The warm-up should be gradual, with heart rate slowly and steadily increasing from Zone 1 to the higher zones, culminating in short repetitions done at or slightly above the expected intensity for the exercise to follow. It should be long enough to prepare you for the intensity of the following activity but not so long as to cause the premature onset of fatigue during the main portion of the workout or in the competition. The length of the warm-up is highly individualized. The warm-up used by a world-class swimmer would completely exhaust a recreational paddler.

To reap the rewards of warm-up, you should complete it within a few minutes of starting the event or main segment of the workout. After about 5 minutes of inactivity the physical benefits of the warm-up are essentially lost.

Just as no warm-up is needed before a low-intensity activity, no cool-down is necessary after a Zone 1 or 2 workout. After a Zone 3 or higher session, however, it is a good idea to continue moving in a sport-specific way, to allow the heart and all the body's other systems to gradually return to a resting level. The cool-down at the end of a workout should be in Zone 1. Research has shown that actively recovering by continuing to move is better than passive recovery, such as merely standing or sitting, as it speeds the removal of waste products from the muscles, reduces body acidity, prevents the pooling of blood in the legs in vertical sports such as running and cross-country skiing, and allows the heart to return safely to a resting state.

The cool-down doesn't need to be long, regardless of the preceding workout's intensity or duration. About 5 to 10 minutes is enough to accomplish all that is physiologically necessary. Longer cool-downs simply use up more precious energy stores, extending the recovery period before your next hard workout. There may be times, however, when extending the cool-down is used to build your aerobic endurance.

[Types of Workouts]

Two broad categories of workouts may be done with your heart rate monitor—steady state and interval. A working knowledge of both will help you understand the heart rate zone workouts that follow this section.

Steady State. This type of workout is the most popular with athletes and the easiest to design, since it involves little or no variation in heart rate once the warm-up is complete. You simply maintain a steady heart rate in your targeted zone. For example, Chapter 4 described AeT workouts in which you maintain a steady heart rate in Zone 2 for an extended period to improve basic aerobic function. This is a good use of steady-state training.

Of course, any targeted heart rate zone may be used for steady-state sessions, but there are limitations on how long the highest zones can be maintained, making this type of workout most effective with the lower heart rate zones. As the target zone and heart rate both rise, the duration of the steady-state portion of a work-

out decreases. While you may do a steady-state workout in Zone 1 for hours, you'll only be able to maintain a steady state for a few minutes in Zone 5b.

Steady-state workouts are excellent for building good endurance and should be a part of every athlete's training regimen. Nearly all workouts in Zones 1 and 2 are steady state. Typically, training for very long events such as Ironman-distance triathlons and ultramarathons is done almost exclusively as steady state, since targeted heart rates are relatively low. As training moves into the higher heart rate zones, though, the workout is generally broken into segments with easy rest breaks, to keep fatigue at bay while increasing the amount of time in the targeted zone. This form of training is called "intervals."

Intervals. Interval training for endurance athletes dates from the early 1900s, but since the 1960s has become increasingly popular. This is considered the most important workout for many high-performance athletes. But while some successful athletes in a number of different sports have used it almost exclusively in their programs, other equally successful athletes seldom do them. Intervals are a potent training tool and can significantly boost your fitness in just a few weeks.

Even the most experienced athletes feel some confusion as to how to conduct an interval session in terms of its intensity. For some, "intervals" simply means short, repeated efforts that are as hard as possible so that you feel like tossing your cookies by the end; for others, intervals are very controlled and structured, using targeted heart rate zones to achieve specific fitness outcomes. Let's take a look at the latter, since throwing up is probably not high on your list of workout objectives.

But first, let's clarify the language used in these workouts. The term "interval" actually refers to the recovery time between hard efforts—*not* to the hard efforts themselves. Yet most athletes use the term in just the opposite way, calling the hard portions the "intervals." To prevent confusion here, we will use the terms *work interval* (WI) and *recovery interval* (RI). As you might suspect, the WI is the part of the interval workout when you're going hard and seeing high heart rates, and the RI is when you're recovering with low heart rates. The RI may be either active recovery (meaning that you continue to run, ride, row, swim, or ski at a low intensity) or passive recovery (meaning essentially that you stop moving altogether, coast, or walk slowly).

Interval workouts generally fall into three categories, based on the energy system they rely on—creatine phosphate, lactic acid, and aerobic.

Creatine phosphate (CP) is a form of energy stored in the muscles that can be accessed quickly and easily, but it burns for only a few seconds. You call on this energy system when doing short, fast sprints. CP intervals are excellent for building muscular power. The WI for these workouts is in the neighborhood of 6 to 12 seconds and done at maximal intensity. Heart rate is not an effective measure for these, since they are so short that your heart doesn't have time to speed up before the WI ends. The RI, on the other hand, is quite long, on the order of 3 to 5 minutes, to allow the body time to produce more CP for the next interval, and may be a combination of passive and active recovery.

On the other end of the interval-duration scale are lengthy workouts done to stress and improve the **aerobic** system. The WI for these are long, 6 to 12 minutes or even more, and the intensity is heart rate Zones 3, 4, and 5a. The RI is generally only about one-fourth as long as the WI's. For example, a 12-minute WI would be followed by a 3-minute RI. These are referred to as "cruise intervals" and are excellent for developing fitness at about the lactate threshold heart rate.

Between the short CP and the long aerobic intervals is the type that most athletes think of when they talk of doing an "interval workout." The body's energy system challenged by this workout is called the **lactic acid** system. It uses glycogen—the body's storage form of carbohydrate—to produce energy. When doing this type of workout, referred to as "anaerobic-endurance" intervals, the intensity is high—well above the LT heart rate in Zone 5b.

Within the category of anaerobic-endurance intervals are two subtypes. The first is effective for developing **aerobic capacity,** or VO_2max— the capacity to use oxygen at a maximum rate during intense exercise. The major determiner of VO_2max is the amount of blood pumped with each beat to the muscles by the heart's left ventricle. It takes a high heart rate (Zone 5b) to challenge and improve the left ventricle's pumping capacity. When forced to work hard, it becomes a more powerful pump in the same way that lifting weights causes your skeletal muscles to become stronger.

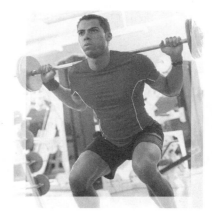

When doing aerobic capacity intervals, the WI is 3 to 5 minutes and done at a heart rate Zone 5b. The RI is active (keep moving) and is equal to the duration of the preceding WI. So following a 3-minute WI, actively recover for 3 minutes. (An exception is swimming, which would have an even shorter RI because of the water's buoyancy, which shortens the recovery time.) A single workout session may include 3 to 5 of these WI. Many athletes can handle 2 such workouts a week as long as they are separated by 48 hours or more.

The second type of anaerobic-endurance intervals is especially good for improving **acid tolerance**—the stuff that causes the burning sensation in your working muscles. Most athletes incorrectly think of this burning as a result of lactic acid. Lactate is actually good for your workout, since it is turned back into energy by the body—it does not cause the stinging. This is a misconception that refuses to go away. The cause of the burning and rapid fatigue is hydrogen ions building up in your body.

You've probably experienced this many times. Whenever you've pushed yourself to the extreme of your limits for just a couple of minutes—say, at your highest heart rates in Zone 5, probably in a race, and quite likely on a hill or trying to stay with a competitor—you've experienced the feeling that you're "blowing up." It's usually accompanied by an uncomfortable sensation in the muscles, perhaps a queasy stomach, and a sense that you may have to slow down significantly or even stop to recover. By doing intervals to improve your tolerance for this hydrogen ion acidity, you can reduce the discomfort and last longer on such efforts.

It's also possible to do **combined-interval** workouts by pairing two or more of these systems into one session. For example, after a good warm-up you could do several 6- to 12-second CP intervals followed by aerobic capacity intervals. Or combine aerobic capacity intervals with cruise intervals. It's best to do the higher-power, more-intense interval portion of the workout first.

Realize that it only takes about 6 to 8 continuous weeks of aerobic capacity intervals to be effective, and 4 to 6 weeks of acid-tolerance intervals. Going beyond these limits means diminished returns and greatly increased risks of injury, overtraining, and burnout. So the bottom line is that you should only employ these workouts in the last few weeks preceding your two or three most important races of the year. That means, at most, doing 24 weeks of aerobic capacity intervals in a year, which is probably too much for most athletes, owing to how stressful they are.

[Workout Structure]

Let's pull all the loose ends from the previous section together to see how a workout is designed. This may sound somewhat simplistic, but understanding a workout's structure will strip away some of the mystery that surrounds training.

A workout is composed of three segments—the warm-up, the mainset, and the cool-down. The mainset is the heart of the workout and is some combination of steady state and intervals. It may include only one of these types or multiple combinations of both. The following are examples of basic workout structures you may use in training:

Example A

- Warm-up
- Mainset—steady state
- Cool-down

Example B

- Warm-up
- Mainset—intervals
- Cool-down

Example C

- Warm-up
- Mainset—intervals + steady state
- Cool-down

Example D

- Warm-up
- Mainset—steady state + intervals + steady state
- Cool-down

Example E

- Warm-up
- Mainset—intervals + steady state + intervals
- Cool-down

The possible combinations are endless. If you are new to your sport, it's best to follow the old K.I.S.S. adage—keep it simple, stupid! Experienced and competitive athletes who fully understand the complexities of their sports and strive to reach their pinnacles of fitness will use many different mainset strategies.

By their very nature, some sports require multiple mainsets. A good example of this is bicycle road racing. Throughout a race a cyclist encounters many changes in velocity and effort, often including some combinations of easy pedaling, all-out sprinting, gut-wrenching hill climbs, time-trial efforts, moderate-effort pack riding, and nice coasting descents. To fully prepare for such an event, the athlete must include many different activities in the mainsets. Using only one mainset strategy won't cut it.

By contrast, some sports, simply by their nature, have much less complex mainsets. Marathon running is a good example of this. The marathoner will do a lot of steady-state mainsets and some intervals. There may even be times when the two are combined to make a single mainset. It is unlikely, however, that the marathoner's training will ever be as complex as that of the cyclist.

Complexity may also come in the form of multiple disciplines making up a mainset, as in triathlon training. This can really get confusing. Not only are there steady state and intervals to think about, but also swimming, biking, and running to throw into the mix. Multisport can be quite a challenge, which may help to explain the rapid growth of the triathlon coaching field in recent years.

The purpose of all training, including intervals, is to prepare the body for competition. With this in mind, your workouts should become increasingly race-like as you approach your most important races. The way that is done is by making the mainsets themselves increasingly like your races, as the season progresses. This has to do with the concept of periodization, which is explored in Chapter 7. Later in this chapter, we'll take a look at mainset combinations.

MAINSETS BY ZONE

Now that you have a handle on the basic structure of zone-targeted workouts—warm-up, mainset, and cool-down—let's examine the details of some suggested zone-workout mainsets. This section will provide just a few examples of these mainsets. The actual number is limited only by your imagination. You can customize the following examples by including hills, cornering, rough water, head wind, high temperature, other athletes, or anything else that may be common to your events. Once you get the hang of it, you can create special mainsets that exactly meet your needs. Look at the following as general guidelines rather than as carved-in-stone ways that all athletes should do each mainset.

[Zone 1: Recovery Mainset]
TYPE: STEADY STATE

TRAINING PURPOSE: This zone is used for easy, recovery-day workouts, warm-ups, and cool-downs. Zone 1 workouts have the potential to hasten recovery from a preceding challenging workout.

PHYSIOLOGICAL BENEFIT: Low-intensity, Zone 1 training places little stress on the muscles while increasing blood flow to them, providing nutrients and oxygen while removing the waste products of preceding hard training sessions.

BE AWARE: Recovery workouts are best used by experienced and fit athletes. If you are new to a sport, you may be better served by not exercising at all rather than training even at Zone 1 intensity on easy days. This is especially true of running, which is an orthopedically stressful sport even for easy workouts. Simply running in Zone 1 the day after a hard workout often leads to injury for novices. Some athletes, especially those over age 50 and those new to endurance sport, may need two or more recovery days following their hardest workouts of the week.

TIMING: Zone 1 workouts are used throughout the year. If you were to graph all your training time by zones for an entire season, Zone 1 would have one of the greatest amounts of likely accumulated time, regardless of the nature of your sport.

> **Example:** Recovery workout. Train steadily in Zone 1 for an extended period, especially on days following high-intensity workouts in Zones 4, 5a, 5b, and 5c.

[Zone 2: Aerobic Threshold Mainsets]
TYPE: STEADY STATE

TRAINING PURPOSE: Zone 2 training improves and maintains basic endurance ability, regardless of the events for which you train. This is the classic "long-distance, slow-distance" zone. For the athlete who participates in events that last 8 to 12 hours, this is race-effort training.

PHYSIOLOGICAL BENEFIT: Working in Zone 2 produces adaptations that improve the athlete's ability to use fat for fuel, while producing shifts in favor of aerobic function by the Type IIa muscle fibers.

BE AWARE: Zone 2 is generally the second most-used intensity, since it is so important to the development of endurance.

TIMING: While Zone 2 workouts should be done year round, they make up a significant part of the athlete's training in the Base period of the season, when improving endurance is a primary objective.

> **Example A:** Low AeT. Exercise steadily in the lower half of Zone 2 for one or more hours, depending on your sport and level of fitness. Observe pace or power, looking for improvements over time at the same heart rates.

> **Example B:** High AeT. Maintain a steady effort in the upper half of Zone 2 for 30 minutes to several hours, depending on your sport and fitness. Building your fitness to be able to maintain this intensity for 1 hour is a minimum recommendation for most endurance sports. For events that are raced entirely in upper Zone 2, the athlete should be able to complete approximately half the anticipated race duration at Zone 2 race intensity in a workout. The upper limit for such a mainset is in the neighborhood of 4 hours, again depending on the sport.

[Zone 3: Tempo Mainsets]
TYPES: STEADY STATE & INTERVAL

TRAINING PURPOSE: Tempo training challenges you to work somewhat hard (RPE 5) with the first indication of heavy breathing, although you are still aerobic. As with Zone 2, the emphasis remains on endurance. The season's first forays into boosting muscular endurance—the ability to maintain a relatively high intensity for a long time (see Chapter 7 for more on muscular endurance)—begins with Zone 3 training. For events lasting approximately 3 to 8 hours, Zone 3 is race effort.

PHYSIOLOGICAL BENEFIT: The Type IIa muscle fibers are maximally challenged in Zone 3, producing a positive change in their aerobic functioning—they become more like slow-twitch, endurance muscle fibers.

BE AWARE: Athletes who participate in events that are not conducted in Zone 3 (events in the 3- to 8-hour range) should limit their Zone 3 time as they approach the race season. The aerobic endurance benefits of Zone 3 workouts are marginally greater than those of upper Zone 2 workouts, but the recovery time in the hours and days afterward is much greater.

TIMING: Zone 3 mainsets are best done in the Base period of the season (see Chapter 7). Those who do Zone 3 events will devote most of their seasons' training to tempo intensity.

> **Example A:** Steady tempo. Train steadily for 20 to 90 minutes in Zone 3. Slowly build from 20 minutes to a longer duration over several weeks. Allow for plenty of recovery in the hours and days following this workout.

> **Example B:** Tempo intervals. Complete 30 to 90 minutes of work intervals that are 12 to 20 minutes in duration, with recovery intervals that are one-fourth as long (for example, following a 12-minute WI, recover for 3 minutes).

[Zone 4: Sub-Lactate Threshold Mainsets]

Type: Steady state and interval.

TRAINING PURPOSE: Training at just below LT improves muscular endurance. It significantly improves performance for events that are about 1 to 3 hours in duration.

PHYSIOLOGICAL BENEFIT: Zone 4 produces changes in the muscles that increase lactate threshold power and pace.

BE AWARE: Training just below LT is an excellent use of training time for the athlete who competes in events lasting 3 hours or less. Going above this intensity level significantly shortens the duration of the effort, because of increasing acidosis.

TIMING: This type of training is best started late in the Base period and continued into the weeks approaching an important event. The durations of the steady-state or work intervals should increase as you build up to an event.

> **Example A:** Cruise intervals. Complete 30 to 60 minutes of intervals that are 6 to 12 minutes long. The recovery intervals are one-fourth the duration of the preceding work interval (for example, following a 6-minute work interval, recover for 90 seconds). When first doing cruise intervals, the work interval durations may descend (such as 12, 10, 8, 6 minutes) to allow for gradual adaptation to longer times at this intensity.
>
> **Example B:** Cruise steady state. Train steadily in Zone 4 for 20 to 30 minutes. This is an advanced workout that is best done following the establishment of good Zone 4 fitness with cruise intervals.

[Zone 5a—Lactate Threshold Mainsets]
TYPE: INTERVAL & STEADY STATE

TRAINING PURPOSE: Muscular endurance is improved by Zone 5a training. Such training forces you to focus on maintaining a steady effort in the face of rapidly increasing discomfort.

PHYSIOLOGICAL BENEFIT: The benefits are the same as for Zone 4, with the addi-

tional benefit of improving your tolerance for accumulating acid in and around the working muscles.

BE AWARE: For the athlete who races in events lasting 20 to 60 minutes, this type of training is critical to success. The recovery time in the hours and days following the workout are somewhat greater than that of Zone 4, because of the anaerobic nature of these workouts.

TIMING: LT Zone workouts are best done in the last 12 weeks or so before important events.

> **Example A:** Cruise intervals. These are the same as Zone 4 intervals, except the intensity builds into Zone 5a as the work interval progresses.
>
> **Example B:** Cruise steady state. Done the same as Zone 4 steady state, but the heart rate and intensity are allowed to increase into Zone 5a in the latter minutes.

[Zone 5b—Aerobic Capacity Mainsets]
TYPE: INTERVAL

TRAINING PURPOSE: Training in Zone 5b improves anaerobic endurance (described in Chapter 7). It is the zone that provides the most effective use of time, if your goal is to race well in events of less than 1 hour's duration. When at the upper end of Zone 5b, you are working at your maximal aerobic capacity.

PHYSIOLOGICAL BENEFIT: Zone 5b boosts aerobic capacity (VO_2max), which is a marker of aerobic fitness by increasing the heart's stroke volume—the amount of blood pumped per beat. This zone also significantly challenges the body's ability to tolerate and remove acid from in and around the working muscles.

BE AWARE: Training in Zone 5b is very stressful for all the body's systems. But that is also why such intensity is so effective for building fitness.

TIMING: For athletes who compete in events of less than 1 hour's duration, Zone 5b workouts are done in the last 12 or so weeks before important competitions. Such workouts may also be done by athletes who race in longer events, but in this case such training is done late in the Base period. This method (which some call "reverse periodization") really is not all that unusual and is discussed in Chapter 8.

> **Example A:** Aerobic capacity intervals. Complete 12 to 20 minutes total of work intervals that are 2 to 4 minutes long. Recovery intervals initially are as long as the preceding work intervals. Over the course of several weeks, shorten the recovery intervals to better simulate the event. As with all interval workouts, at the completion of this mainset you should feel as if you could have done one more work interval.

> **Example B:** 30-30s. Alternate 30 seconds at aerobic capacity effort, pace, or power (heart rate responds too slowly to be effective for gauging intensity) with 30 seconds at recovery effort, pace, or power. Build to about 24 such intervals over 3 to 4 weeks. Be careful not to make the intensity higher than Zone 5b early in the workout. If you fade in the last few intervals, you probably started out too fast.

[Zone 5c–Anaerobic Capacity Mainsets]
TYPE: INTERVAL

TRAINING PURPOSE: Zone 5c training prepares the athlete for those rare (for most

sports) seconds in a race when a maximal output decides the outcome.

PHYSIOLOGICAL BENEFIT: Zone 5c develops muscular power while maximally challenging the body's tolerance for and removal of acid from in and around the working muscles.

BE AWARE: Few endurance sports require such intensity. An exception is road cycling, which often comes down to a sprint at the end of the race. Most endurance athletes should not do these workouts. Heart rate is not a good indicator of Zone 5c intensity, owing to how short the work intervals are. Intensity is best monitored by RPE, pace, or power. The recovery from Zone 5c workouts is extensive. The risk of injury is also high when doing these workouts.

TIMING: Zone 5c training is best done in the last 8 to 12 weeks before important races.

> **Example A:** CP intervals. The purpose of this mainset is to improve your body's capacity for power development and to enhance its ability to recover by generating more creatine phosphate following sprints. Once every 5 minutes of the mainset, do a maximum-effort (RPE 10) for 8 to 15 seconds. Do not allow good form to be compromised. If you begin to get sloppy or if power or velocity fades, stop the mainset and begin the cool-down. Do as many as 15 of these in a mainset. You may break the intervals into sets of 3 to 5 work intervals, each with 10 minutes of recovery between sets. Again, do not continue if form begins to break down.

> **Example B:** Hydrogen stacker. Be forewarned: This mainset creates extremely high levels of acidosis and is a painful experience you won't want to repeat too often. However, if you do short but

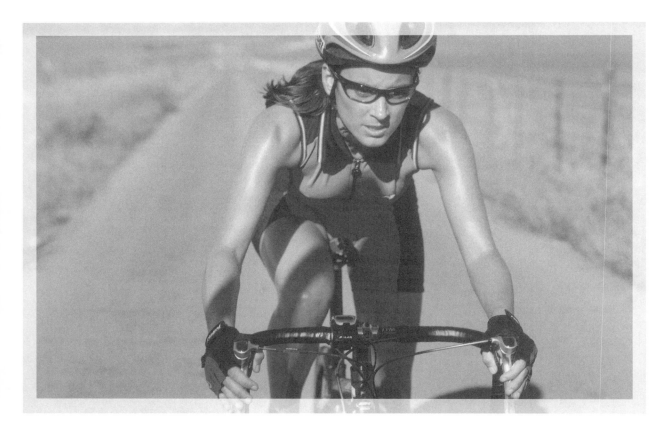

fast endurance events, such as bicycle criterium racing, this mainset will develop the capacity to remove and buffer acid, allowing you to continue pushing the effort. Here is how it's done: Do 4, 20- to 40-second, near-maximum-effort (RPE 10) sprints with 20-second recovery intervals. That counts as 1 set. Do 1 to 3 such sets in a mainset, with 5 minutes of very easy recovery (passive and active) between sets. The duration of the work intervals and the number of sets depends on the demands of the event for which you are training. Start at the low end of each, and add duration and sets as your fitness improves. **Do not do this workout unless you are an experienced and extremely fit athlete with a low risk for cardiovascular disease.** It is

highly stressful. One of these in a week is plenty. Allow at least 72 hours for recovery afterward.

COMBINED **MAINSETS**

Each of the above mainset examples represents one portion of a mainset. A workout usually only has one portion to its mainset. But, as described above, you may combine two or more of them into a mainset to create an advanced workout that closely simulates the demands of the events for which you train, to add variety to your workouts, or simply to save you time.

The following are some common mainset combinations. It may be necessary to reduce the number or duration of intervals, or the duration of a steady state, to make these workouts more manageable, especially early in the season when your fitness might not allow you to handle a lot of workload. These combined workouts are *only* for experienced athletes. Novices should strictly use single-mainset workouts.

[Common Mainset Combinations]

- Cruise Intervals + Low AeT
- Aerobic Capacity Intervals + Cruise Intervals
- 30-30s + Cruise Steady State
- Tempo Intervals + High AeT
- 30-30s + Cruise Intervals + Steady Tempo
- CP Intervals + Aerobic Capacity Intervals + CP Intervals

Each endurance sport has unique demands—not only for the way the mainset portions may be combined and arranged, but also for other details, such as cadence or body position. Feel free to modify these mainsets or to create altogether new ones that better fit the distinctive characteristics of your sport.

COMPETITION ZONES

If you train to compete in races, heart rate can serve as a handy governor for how hard to work during the event. In steady-state events such as running races and triathlons, knowing how high you can push the effort gives you the freedom to work hard but not so hard as to cause the onset of early fatigue. If your pacing is just right, you will cross the finish line strongly but totally wasted, knowing you gave it everything you had. If you go too hard, at some point

in the race you will "blow up" and have to slow down dramatically, losing more time than had you stayed with a more conservative pace. This is most likely to happen early in the race as a result of excitement and a sense of being "bullet proof." Almost every athlete in every race goes out too fast at the start…and pays for it later with great suffering and decreased velocity.

While heart rate can help you avoid this dilemma, it is still important to have a pacing strategy and stick with it. This strategy is based on information—not only your heart rate but also pace or power, since heart rate responds slowly in the first few minutes even though the velocity may be high. So here's another handy reference point. In mass start, steady-state events, such as a marathon, you can assume that everyone around you will start too fast. Let them go. Others should be passing you for the first several minutes. If they aren't—you *also* went out too fast and will pay for this mistake later on.

Once you settle into the proper race pace or power, heart rate will gradually increase and then level out, indicating effort. This will help you to gauge and make decisions about velocity for the rest of the competition. In general, we can say that for any given steady state–event duration there is an associated heart rate range that is right for you. The key to proper race pacing, then, is to discover that heart rate range. This is one of the reasons we train—to learn how the body responds to racelike effort. From your training you should be able to narrow your heart rate range to something that is appropriate for the conditions of the event and your level of fitness. Table 5.1 can help you with that process.

EVENT DURATION	ZONE
>12 hours	1
8–12 hours	2
3–8 hours	3
1–3 hours	4
20 minutes–1 hour	5a
2–20 minutes	5b
<2 minutes	5c

Table 5.1. Suggested Heart Rate Zones to Target for Steady-State Events by Event Duration

The table suggests a heart rate zone that should be about right for a steady-state event that you will likely complete in a given amount of time. The trickiest part is those events that you will complete in a time that is on the borderline, such as in running a marathon in just under 3 hours. Should you be in the upper Zone 3 or in lower Zone 4? The only way to answer that question is by training at the targeted pace and seeing how your heart rate responds. That will give you enough information to make a decision so that you can use heart rate wisely to help you make pacing decisions during the race, such as "Am I going too fast?" or "Could I go faster?"

THE **HEART** OF THE **MATTER**

This chapter guided you through the details of designing a workout. You learned that a workout has three components—the warm-up, the mainset, and the cool-down. Heart rate may be used to guide intensity through each segment.

Zone I is used in both the warm-up and the cool-down, which are essentially mirror images—heart rate rises in the warm-up and drops in the cool-down. The mainset—the heart of the workout—is made up either of a steady state or intervals, or both. You can use heart rate zones in many ways when doing steady-state and interval workouts. The higher the targeted zone, the more likely it is that you will use intervals, as it becomes increasingly difficult to maintain the effort for long enough periods of time to produce total fitness, especially when exercising in Zones 5a, 5b, and 5c.

Heart rate is also beneficial when preparing for a steady-state race. Race intensity may be determined for goal performance times, based on zones. Once the goal zone is decided, you can train at that intensity in getting ready for the race. Then, in the race, heart rate will prevent you from going too fast and will keep you on track for a successful event outcome.

Having read this chapter, you should now have a good grasp of how to use heart rate to govern the stress of workouts and races. The next chapter takes this one step farther by introducing a system of training that uses your heart rate monitor.

6

THE TRAINING TRIAD AND HEART RATE

To many athletes, training is random—a hodgepodge of disconnected workouts. Every day when it's time to work out, they simply do whatever pops into their heads. It's as much entertainment as training. Their fitness-building programs are little more than collections of often-repeated exercise sessions done without logic, pattern, or purpose. But the body is a remarkable mechanism and, despite this lack of focus, fitness still improves for a while. The problem is that the resulting fitness may not be what is needed for the targeted event. For example, the fitness required to run a 5k road race is far different from that necessary for a marathon. Another problem with random training is that fitness plateaus early in the season, once the body adapts to the same old repetitive stress.

These problems are easily fixed. All it takes is an understanding of, and use of, a proven training methodology—plus the dedication to follow through with it. Having a purpose and a plan for each workout is really not difficult. This chapter will show you how by providing a sound structure for your heart rate–based training.

THE TRAINING TRIAD

In the 1970s I was a young man intent on becoming the best athlete possible. I believed that to achieve this I needed a better understanding of training, so I returned to the university to start a program in exercise science. I soon discovered that although my professors knew the science of training, at least what there was to know in that era, when it came to application in the real world they didn't have a clue. After three years I came away from the university with a master's degree in science—and a lot more questions than answers. I still did not understand the application of training science. I came to realize that if I could draw a comprehensive diagram of training, one that was simple and yet summarized all there was to know about training, I could organize all the science I recently learned and get a firm grasp of how to apply it to a real athlete—namely, me. My search for this "holy grail" began in 1978.

I played around with various diagrams trying to find the key. Maybe training is unidirectional and could be represented by a straight line, I thought. Or maybe it is a circle, with a never-ending repetition of certain activities. Or perhaps it has three dimensions, like a spiral. None of this took me anywhere. Then in the early 1980s I came across a book—*The Theory and Methodology of Training* by Tudor Bompa, Ph.D., a former Romanian sports scientist who now lives in Canada and continues teaching at York University, consulting with national sports federations and speaking widely. Here I found what I was looking for—and it was beautifully simple. Eventually, I was able to meet with Dr. Bompa and pick his brain about my elusive diagram and much of what was presented in his book. We have continued to stay in contact over many years.

In his groundbreaking book Dr. Bompa, now often referred to as "the Father of Periodization," presented the concept of biomotor abilities by using a simple triangle. When I saw this graphic I knew I had finally found the diagram that was my key to understanding training application. I have used that figure ever since in training athletes. I call it the "Training Triad."

It is a simple figure, but I soon came to realize that there was much to be learned from it. The Triad not only illustrates the activities that make up what we call "training," but also suggests the sequence in which the training activities are scheduled into an athlete's single season as well as when planning one's career.

It all starts with understanding the performance abilities you are trying to improve as end products of training. These abilities are illustrated by Figure 6.1. Understanding the concepts related to the Training Triad will simplify the complexities of training by removing much of the guesswork.

What this figure shows us is that there are six physical abilities related to performance regardless of the sport. They are as follows:

- *Endurance*—the ability to maintain a relatively low level of intensity for a long time.

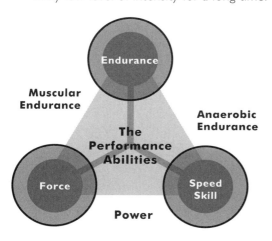

Fig. 6.1. The Training Triad

- *Force*—the ability to overcome environmental resistance such as gravity, water, or wind.
- *Speed Skill*—the ability to make the movements of the sport in an economical manner at the required cadence.
- *Muscular Endurance*—the ability to maintain a moderately high level of force for a relatively long time.
- *Anaerobic Endurance*—the ability to maintain a high level of speed skill while working at a near-maximal effort for a relatively long time.
- *Power*—the ability to produce a high level of force with a high level of speed skill.

Again, it doesn't matter what sport we are talking about here. It could be endurance sports such as running, cycling, and rowing, or power sports like football, basketball, and baseball. It simply makes no difference at all. Training for *any* sport is made up of some unique mix of each of these same six abilities. Generally, endurance sports favor the abilities in the upper half of the figure—endurance, muscular endurance, and anaerobic endurance—while power sports rely mostly on the abilities in the lower half—power, force, and speed skill. But each sport requires some level of contribution from all of these six abilities.

The abilities at the corners of the Triad are the *basic abilities*—endurance, force, and speed skill. Those on the sides of the Triad are the *advanced abilities*—muscular endurance, anaerobic endurance, and power. Each uniquely contributes to athletic performance, and each is developed through training in a special manner. Heart rate provides important information to help you develop and use each of the abilities.

	ENDURANCE	FORCE	SPEED SKILL
Description	Long, low- to moderate-intensity distance	Resisted efforts (gravity, water, wind)	Short repeats emphasizing form
Primary Benefit	Cardiorespiratory system	Muscular system	Nervous system
Intensity	Zone 2	Zones 3 & 4	Greater than race effort (too brief for heart rate response)
Workout Example	Maintain steady effort for 1 hour	Train on hilly course, working hard on uphills	6 x 20-sec. fast reps with 80-sec. recoveries

Table 6.1. Summary of the Basic Abilities

THE BASIC ABILITIES

Regardless of sport, level of accomplishment, competitiveness, experience, age, or gender, all athletes must fully develop their basic abilities. To neglect these in favor of training the more challenging advanced abilities means you will never even come close to your potential as an endurance athlete. Creating a high level of fitness in the basic abilities is always necessary for exceptional performance. Endurance athletes generally do a good job of building the endurance ability, but many are lacking when it comes to force and speed skill.

Those who are new to their sport should spend nearly all their training time for the first year or two focused on the basic abilities. These are slow to develop and require a long period of concentrated training. Endurance is especially slow to respond, as many physiological changes are necessary in the development of this ability.

The experienced athlete will return to the basic abilities every year for a few weeks at the start of the training season and may come back to them again from time to time throughout the season. Even when not focused on developing these three abilities, the seasoned athlete will maintain their fitness. Ability maintenance, a unique aspect of training, will be discussed later in this chapter.

For now let's get a better grasp of what each of the basic abilities is about and how you can use your heart rate monitor in their development. Table 6.1 summarizes the key elements of each one.

[Endurance]

This is probably the type of training with which you are most familiar. After all, endurance training is the foundation of all endurance sports. Training to improve endurance is based on doing long workouts ("long" being relative to the event for which you are training) at a low to moderate effort. The primary physiological benefit of such training is the improvement of the heart, lungs, and blood in their contribution to endurance performance. These workouts are carried out at or slightly above the aerobic threshold, as described in Chapter 4. This is heart rate Zone 2. Examples of such training sessions from Chapter 5 are the "low-AeT" and "high-AeT" workouts.

[Force]

If you are an endurance athlete, you probably are not quite comfortable with the idea of force training. But if you were a weight lifter, this ability would make perfect sense. In force workouts some sort of resistance is applied that the body must overcome. This resistance can be in the form of gravity, as when going uphill or the drag caused by water or wind. It can also be some sort of tethering device, as in swimming. When you do force workouts the purpose is to improve the strength of muscle. Every athlete, including those in endurance sports, requires some level of muscular strength for high-level performance. Endurance athletes tend to shy away from certain types of force training—usually weight lifting—because of a concern that they will become bulky. That's unlikely, with a strength program designed for endurance sport, but that's a topic for a different book.

Common ways for endurance athletes to develop force are by training on hills and by increasing the drag of water or wind with baggy clothing or even with drag devices such as parachutes. Running or riding a bike uphill causes your muscles to work harder to overcome the resistance of gravity. That's why your heart rate rises on hills. This is a great way to improve the force of your muscles.

Years ago when I coached a masters swim group we did a "force workout" once a week in which the athletes swam wearing a T-shirt to increase the resistance of the water. It made them stronger. Greater ability to overcome resistance means improved performance in your endurance sport.

It's necessary to raise the intensity of these workouts above that used for endurance training in order to challenge the muscles, but avoid exceeding the lactate threshold. This means exercising in heart rate Zones 3 and 4.

[Speed Skill]

With some sport exceptions, notably swimming, this is the ability most neglected by endurance athletes. We tend not to think of the nervous system when building greater fitness. But it is every bit as important as the body's other systems when it comes to performance. If nervous system training is avoided, the athlete wastes precious energy from poor technique. Yet most endurance athletes think they have good, if not excellent, technique. And if not perfect, they believe tinkering with technique will cause even greater problems. They are wrong.

It is common to see runners who land on their heels and bound with a slow cadence, cyclists whose bike position and poor pedaling technique rob them of energy, rowers who drag or fail to "feather" the oar on recovery, swimmers who "fishtail," and cross-country skiers who don't complete the push phase before starting to glide. Endurance athletes who waste energy and who experience premature fatigue as a result of poor technique will never come close to their sport potential. Energy conservation through technique improvement should be a high priority for every endurance athlete and regularly included in training.

The type of workout done to improve speed skills involves short repeats, with an emphasis on perfect form. "Short" in this case generally means less than 30 seconds. There should be a relatively long recovery—30 to 90 seconds—between these repeats to ensure that the body is fully recovered before doing the next one. When fatigue begins to set in, to even a very small degree, speed skill training will no longer be effective. You cannot adequately train the nervous system if the body is tiring. Sloppiness sets in. So these workouts are best kept short but done frequently. The higher the frequency of speed skill workouts in training, the more rapid will be the improvement.

Speed skill workouts are unique in that heart rate is not a good indicator of intensity since the duration of the repeats is so brief. Heart rate just doesn't have a chance to "catch up" and tell you how hard you are working. Perceived exertion, pace, and power are better intensity indicators for speed skill workouts.

Examples of this type of training are what runners call "strides," cyclists call isolated leg training, and swimmers do as drills.

THE ADVANCED ABILITIES

Once the basic abilities are developed, it's time to go to work on the advanced abilities—muscular endurance, anaerobic endurance, and power. These are the abilities that determine high-level performance in endurance events for competitive athletes. But if finishing the race is your main concern, then your training must focus solely on the basic abilities. Training of the advanced abilities is strictly intended for experienced and well-conditioned athletes who are intent on performing at or near their potential for their chosen sport.

Compared with the basic abilities, the advanced abilities respond quickly to training. Even for the seasoned veteran, it takes months at the start of the training year to reestablish high levels of endurance, force, and speed skill. But a high level of advanced-ability fitness can be achieved in only a few weeks, although these abilities respond at different rates. Most athletes find that muscular endurance comes around more slowly than anaerobic endurance, which responds more slowly than power. In other words, power can be built quickly in just a matter of a few workouts, with the other two lagging not far behind.

Each of the advanced abilities is the resultant of the basic abilities at its adjoining corners. For example, to create exceptional muscular endurance first requires that you develop exceptional endurance and force. If endurance and force are not fully developed first, then regardless of how much muscular endurance training is done it will fall well short of your potential. This is why you must concentrate on the basic abilities early in the training season before beginning to train the advanced abilities.

Just as with the basic abilities, your heart rate monitor is a great tool to help you build the high-performance advanced abilities. Let's examine the details more closely. Table 6.2 summarizes the advanced abilities and how heart rate is used in their improvement.

[Muscular Endurance]

Regardless of your sport, if you are an endurance athlete you know that muscular

	MUSCULAR ENDURANCE	ANAEROBIC ENDURANCE	POWER
Description	Long, moderate intervals with short recoveries, or long, steady efforts	Short, fast intervals with about equal recoveries	Very short, very fast intervals with long recoveries
Primary Benefit	Lactate threshold pace and power	Aerobic capacity pace and power	Muscle fiber recruitment
Intensity	Zones 3–5a	Zone 5b	Zone 5c (or all-out effort)
Workout Example (see Chapter 5)	Cruise intervals	Aerobic capacity intervals	CP intervals

Table 6.2. Summary of the Advanced Abilities

endurance (ME) plays a pivotal role in your performance. As you build a higher level of ME, your pace or power at lactate threshold improves, as do all efforts slightly below this pace or power. When endurance athletes have top-drawer ME, they often say they feel "strong." This means they feel as if they can hold a fairly high velocity or power for a long time. They often finish the race and say they could have kept on going. While they lack truly high-end velocity, their abundance of ME means races feel almost easy, so long as the pace or power changes very little.

Two type of workouts are common in ME training—long-duration, steady efforts and long intervals with short recoveries. These workouts are done in Zones 3, 4, and 5a. One type of ME workout previously described in Chapter 5 is "steady tempo." In this workout you train steadily for 20 to 90 minutes in Zone 3, building from the shorter to the longer duration over several weeks.

Another example of a higher-intensity ME workout from Chapter 5 was "cruise intervals,"

done in Zones 4 and 5a. You may recall that these work intervals are 6 to 12 minutes long with recovery intervals that are one-fourth the duration of the preceding work interval. An example is 4, 8-minute work intervals with 2-minute recoveries. A total of 30 to 60 minutes of accumulated work interval time is done in a single session.

[Anaerobic Endurance]

This type of workout is most effective if you compete in events that last less than 1 hour, although anaerobic endurance (AE) is also effective for advanced athletes who compete in longer events. The primary benefit of AE training is an increase of your aerobic capacity (VO_2 max)—the physiological capability to use oxygen to produce maximal work. With an increase in aerobic capacity, there is a "trickle-down" effect that benefits all submaximal efforts.

Zone 5b is the target heart rate when AE is the workout goal. When at the upper end of Zone 5b, you are working at or very near your maximal aerobic capacity. This makes such train-

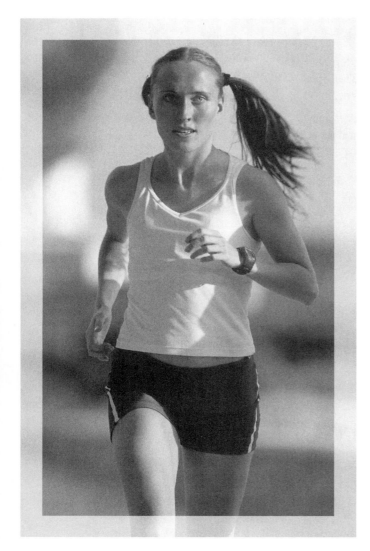

recovery period that may last several days for some athletes.

The type of workout used for AE training involves fast work intervals of a few minutes' duration with recovery intervals that are about equal in duration. An example of this is "aerobic capacity intervals." As described in Chapter 5, this workout involves completing a total of 12 to 20 minutes of work intervals at Zone 5b that are 2 to 4 minutes long. The recovery intervals are also 2 to 4 minutes, depending on the length of the work interval. In the initial few seconds or even minutes of the first work interval, heart rate will respond slowly, so you need to use a rating of perceived exertion to get the pacing or power right until heart rate "catches up." With each subsequent work interval, heart rate will respond more quickly, decreasing the amount of time needed to estimate proper output. As with all interval workouts, at the completion of this mainset you should feel as if you could have done one more work interval.

[Power]

The ability to produce a great amount of power quickly is critical to success in events such as bicycle road races, which often come down to an all-out sprint for the finish line. The athlete who can recruit the most muscle the quickest is a good bet to win. Understanding this muscle recruitment requires knowing a bit of physiology.

Assume that you are picking up a light object, such as this book, with one hand and curling it toward your shoulder as the elbow bends. It won't take much effort to do that, and so you will use slow-only twitch muscle fibers (Type I) since it doesn't "cost" the body much to use them. The book is easily curled using only

ing a powerful tool, since aerobic capacity plays an important role in endurance performance. One series of research studies on this type of training, coming out of a lab in Paris, found that it improved not only aerobic capacity but also lactate threshold pace, while it enhanced speed skill.

Although AE training is a very powerful workout, you must be careful in its application, as it is also stressful and requires an extensive

Type I muscles. But if you make the movement with a slightly heavier object, the brain will ask more muscle fibers for help and so next calls on some unique fibers—the ones that have both slow- and fast-twitch characteristics (Type IIa), discussed earlier in Chapter 4. If the object is *really* heavy, the brain knows that it will take more than Type I and Type IIa to curl the object and so it asks for Type IIb—the pure fast-twitch muscle fibers—to help out. This use-all-we've-got recruitment pattern is common for all movement that demands maximum effort in a minimal time, such as sprinting. The athlete who can recruit all these fibers in the least amount of time and maintain their near-maximal output the longest, usually only a few seconds, wins the sprint.

If your races are often determined by such sprinting and you want to be competitive, then training your power ability is necessary. Again, this is only for advanced athletes.

Chapter 5 introduced you to creatine phosphate (CP) intervals. These are excellent for teaching your body to quickly recruit muscle fibers. The work interval is quite short—about 6 to 12 seconds—and done at maximal intensity. The key to this workout is rapid recruitment of muscle fibers. From the first stride or stroke use all the muscle fibers you can call on instantaneously. When fatigue begins to set in you will no longer be able to recruit quickly, and so the part of the workout dedicated to power must end. Continuing to do these intervals when you can no longer get the Type IIb fibers to respond is more than a waste of time. It also teaches your body to avoid using Type IIb.

Heart rate is not effective when doing CP intervals, they are so brief that the heart begins to speed up only when the interval ends. But that's not a big deal since you are attempting an all-out effort and not holding back or pacing yourself at all. The recovery after each work interval is relatively long, about 3 to 5 minutes, so that the body can restore its energy-rich CP and get ready for the next interval. Your heart rate should drop to very low levels during each recovery.

THE HEART OF THE MATTER

There are six abilities that define what training is all about for the endurance athlete—endurance, force, speed skill, muscular endurance, anaerobic endurance, and power. Each plays an important role in performance and is improved through training in a unique way. For most of them, heart rate is an excellent tool for ensuring that you get the intensity for each right, in order to reap the benefits of the workouts.

While this chapter was all about training with intensity, the next one is about making sure you don't overdo it. Too much of a good thing can ruin your season.

7

BALANCING REST AND STRESS

This book has used the word "fitness" a lot without defining it. I'm sure you've got a good handle on what the word means when it comes to your sport. You may know, for example, that if your event is timed and steady state, such as running a 10k race, producing a certain time means you are fit. You may even know what it takes in the way of training to reach that level of fitness. If you participate in variably paced events like bicycle road races, you know that if you can stay with the leaders when the pace picks up and still be with them at the finish, then you are fit. It may be helpful, however, to look at the concept of fitness in a way you may never have thought of before. It is this—that fitness may be defined by a simple formula:

Fitness = rest − stress

To improve your fitness, the training must be stressful enough to give your body a "reason" to grow stronger. If the workout is too easy, your body won't change, as it has no need to do so. It adapts only if the demands placed on it are greater than what it can currently handle. This doesn't mean that all workouts should be stressful. Some should be easy (Zone 1) to permit rest and recovery.

In the long term, though, properly balancing the two producers of fitness—rest and stress—essentially means that when you subtract stress from rest there is something left over. In other words, the amount of rest should exceed the amount of stress in your training.

Balancing rest and stress is much like managing a checking account to make sure you don't run out of money. Writing a check may be compared with exercising. The check you write (workout) can be a large one or a small one. Making an account deposit is similar to resting. You can make a big or little deposit (rest). What you *don't* want to do is have your checking account in a negative balance for too long. If you write a big check and don't make a big enough deposit to cover it, you will be penalized by the bank with a hefty fee. In the case of your body this penalty is called "overtraining," which is discussed later in this chapter.

You may know, however, that you can have your checking account overdrawn in your check register for a couple of days, so long as you make a deposit soon. Again, it's the same with your body—you can overtrain for a few days and, so long as you soon make an adequate deposit in the form of rest, your body will be "in the black" once again with no penalty.

This chapter discusses how to use both stress and rest to create a high level of fitness without becoming overtrained. You'll learn to make fatigue your friend, build a high level of fitness using the short-term power of overtraining, and measure the stress of workouts and entire weeks of training using your heart rate monitor.

OPTIMIZING STRESS AND REST

Your heart rate monitor is a great tool for monitoring and regulating workout stress. It tells you not only how hard the workout is but also what your body is experiencing in terms of stress from other sources such as heat, emotions, dehydration, and even the onset of illness. Knowing that heart rate is an indicator of total stress helps you to make informed decisions about exercise. The most basic decision to be made is how hard to make the workout on any given day.

[Increasing Stress]

Over the course of several weeks, as you approach an A-priority event, the stress applied to the body in the form of exercise should become increasingly like the goal event's targeted intensity. This usually means increasing the intensity of workouts as the season progresses. It's important that this workout stress increases gradually over the course of the season. You cannot "force" the body to become more fit. Trying to do that will ultimately lead to breaking down in some way.

It is always best to gently coax the body to higher levels of fitness by gradually raising both

WEEKS	EMPHASIS ZONE	MAINTAIN ZONES
4	2	–
4	3	2
4	4–5a	2
4	5b	2, 4–5a
4	5c	2, 4–5a, 5b

Table 7.1. Seasonal Heart Rate Zone Training Progression for Short or Variably Paced Events

WEEKS	EMPHASIS ZONE	MAINTAIN ZONES
4	2	–
4	3	2
4	4–5a	2
4	5b	2, 4–5a
8	2	4–5a, 5b

Table 7.2. Seasonal Heart Rate Zone Training Progression for Long (8+ Hours) Endurance Events

the heart rate zones and the time spent in the higher zones over a long period. Many changes must happen at the cellular level for fitness to improve, and these cannot be hurried. It's difficult, if not impossible, to say what that time schedule should look like for any given person, considering how we are each unique. But a general guideline is to stay with one heart rate zone for 4 weeks before starting to train in the next higher zone. Doing this allows the body to adapt slowly and safely, which builds "deeper" fitness than if the training is rushed. Such a progression would look something like Table 7.1 for the athlete who participates in short, fast events:

While the seasonal heart rate zone training progression may look like what is presented in this table for those doing short events such as 5k and 10k running or cross-country ski races and 1500-meter swims, or variably paced events such as mass-start bicycle races, this progression is not meant for all events. Preparing for long endurance events such as an Ironman triathlon might look something like what is shown in Table 7.2.

[Balancing Stress with Rest]

For the serious athlete, the key to successful training is frequently stressing the body with challenging workouts at the higher heart rate zones or over long periods in lower zones. The more often these harder workouts can be done—assuming adequate rest is provided—the greater the athlete's fitness becomes in a given period of time. The most important key to quick recovery is adequate rest. So how can you ensure that you get enough rest to recover promptly from workout fatigue? The next section addresses this.

FATIGUE, RECOVERY, AND FITNESS

Let's clear up one misconception before we go any further—exercise stress does *not* create fitness. Exercise only creates the *potential* for fitness. Fitness is not realized until you rest following exercise. The best type of rest is sleep, for it's during sleep that the body releases growth hormone to build a more fit body. The sidebar "Growth Hormone" on page 90 explains this remarkable hormone and its benefits for fitness.

What exercise *does* create is fatigue. We tend to view fatigue as the foe that must be defeated and removed. But that will never happen—and you wouldn't want it to. Fatigue is there to stop you from doing damage to the body. Without it you might exercise to the point of tearing muscles, fracturing bones, and even killing yourself. Fatigue is like your friendly, neighborhood police officer—you never want it to go away completely. What you want to do, though, is to keep the officer away until he is really needed. You don't want a cop hanging around all the time—only when you are in trouble and at risk for being hurt. That's when fatigue should step in and protect you.

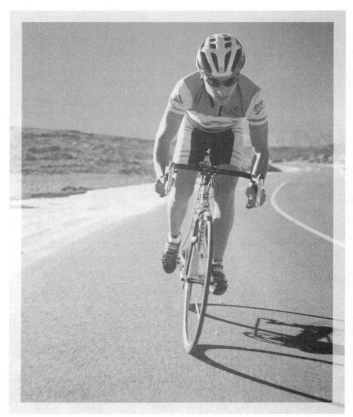

GROWTH HORMONE

Training long and hard isn't enough. Reaching your best possible performance in sport also requires chemistry, especially the body's hormones. When it comes to improving fitness, human growth hormone is one of the driving forces that makes all the hard work pay off.

Without growth hormone (GH), all your training would be wasted time, because your body would not respond with greater fitness. Maintaining, or even increasing, natural levels of GH has a positive effect on athletic performance. So what can you do to stimulate GH? Before answering that question, let's examine GH more closely.

GH is secreted by the marble-sized pituitary gland at the base of the brain, and has an anabolic effect. You've probably heard of the illegal use of "anabolic steroids" and know what that means for performance. Natural GH provides some of the same benefits—promotion of muscle growth and reductions in body fat—without the negative consequences.

GH is released in pulses during and immediately following exercise, and especially during sleep. Peak levels of GH are attained during puberty, and begin a steady decline at about age 25. After age 30, GH falls off about 14 percent for each successive decade of life. For example, at age 20, peak value may be 500 micrograms (mcg), drop to 200 mcg at 40, and sink to 25 mcg by age 80. So the older you are, the more important it is to promote GH production.

Of course, another route is always available to those who want to pay the price. Synthetic GH is available for medical treatment of conditions such as failure to grow in children, and for recovery following surgery. Some athletes have been suspected of using synthetic GH, which is banned by the International Olympic Committee and a variety of national organizations.

Maintaining or boosting natural levels of GH to promote rapid recovery of muscles and other tissues, reduce body fat, and maintain immune system function is possible by monitoring diet and exercise. Recent research has found all the following to be effective for increasing GH levels:

- **Dietary fat.** Eating fat, especially monounsaturated (olive oil, nuts, avocados) and saturated (meats), promotes GH production. Polyunsaturated fats (vegetable oils), however, appear to have a negative effect on GH levels.

- **Protein.** As protein in the diet goes up, GH production declines. Taking in protein immediately after exercise along with carbohydrate, however, seems to improve GH levels.

- **Exercise intensity.** Exercising in Zone 5 causes the pituitary gland to release more GH than does exercising in the lower heart rate zones.

- **Workload variety.** One study found that maintaining a constant level of exercise workload for 3 weeks resulted in a leveling off of the body's GH production.

Based on current information, it looks as if the best ways to promote performance-boosting GH levels are to eat adequate levels of dietary fat, take in protein along with carbohydrate following workouts, occasionally train in Zone 5, and increase the training workload every 3 weeks or so.

[What Is Fatigue?]

Fatigue during exercise is not as simple as it seems on the surface. The cause varies with the intensity and duration of exercise. In a 20-minute event in which you are working in Zone 5b, you fatigue for a different reason than if doing a 10-hour event with heart rate in Zone 2. Fatigue is caused by several things. Other than overheating and dehydration that can slow or stop your exercise, there are at least four common physiological causes of fatigue during endurance events that are generally accepted by sports science:

Increasing body acidity. Hydrogen ions accumulate in and around the hard-working muscles. Such fatigue is common in steady-state events lasting less than 1 hour and in the highest intensity moments in variably paced events when heart rate is in Zones 5a, 5b, or 5c. It is marked by heavy, labored breathing and a burning sensation in the working limbs (legs or arms). There is a feeling that you are "redlined." Workouts done in Zone 5 prepare the body for this kind of fatigue by producing buffers to offset the acid and by removing the hydrogen ions from the body.

Depletion of muscle glycogen. This is the body's storage form of carbohydrate. Glycogen is a limited fuel source. Your body only has enough stored for about 90 to 120 minutes of intense exercise. If you don't replace it by using a sports drink or something similar in events lasting longer than about an hour, then you will begin to feel tired and heavy and find it difficult to continue. You will feel an overwhelming desire to stop moving. Many sports refer to this sensation as "bonking."

Neuromuscular junction failure. The nervous system transmits electrochemical impulses from the spinal cord to the muscle fiber. Where the nerve axon meets the muscle fiber is where the muscle innervations occur. This stimulation late in an exercise session may fail, for some unknown reason. When it does, the athlete is unable to fully stimulate a muscle group to contract, resulting in what may be called fatigue. This may also be associated with cramping. Neuromuscular junction failure may occur in events of any duration or heart rate intensity. Since this fatigue type is not fully understood, how to avoid it is something of a mystery. The possibilities include being adequately hydrated, eating a diet rich in electrolytes, and having a high level of fitness relative to the event in which you are competing.

Increase of tryptophan in the brain. We don't know a lot about this fatigue factor either. Here's what is known. In long-duration events, usually on the order of 3 hours or more with intensity in the lower zones, certain changes take place in the blood amino acid levels. These changes lead to subtle chemical reactions that increase tryptophan levels in the brain, causing you to feel lethargic and sleepy (tryptophan is what helps you go to sleep at night). You may yawn, feel like lying down, and even have trouble keeping your eyes open. Merely finishing becomes a struggle. You probably can't train to prevent this type of fatigue. If you typically experience these fatigue symptoms, it may help to supplement your diet with branched chain amino acids before the exercise session begins.

[Hard-Easy Cycles]

What is described above is short-term fatigue that happens during exercise. But there is also long-term fatigue, whose biological causes are not fully understood. The cause may be as simple as chronically low levels of glycogen, or as complex as neuromuscular or hormonal shifts. This type of fatigue will accumulate over time if allowed to go unchecked. The way to avoid this is to follow the principle of hard-easy training cycles.

Hard training days—meaning high heart rate zones or long-duration workouts in low heart rate zones—should be followed by easy days. Easy days are those with short workouts done in heart rate Zone 1, or days with no exercise at all. In the same way, a few weeks of hard training should be followed by some easy days. Several months of hard training are best concluded with a number of easy weeks. The details of these hard-easy cycles are described in detail in Chapter 8.

OVERTRAINING—WHEN MORE MEANS LESS

The smart athlete includes enough volume and intensity in training sessions to create stress, with some fatigue resulting in the hours afterward. A little fatigue is a good thing because it means that greater fitness will soon occur—if enough easy training or time off from exercise follows. But what all too often happens is that the athlete decides to do more, and the fatigue becomes insidious. If the athlete continues to push the hard training while ignoring the need for rest, overtraining sets in.

Most of us have a simplistic view of overtraining, thinking that we merely did a little too much exercise and therefore we're tired. There's much more to it than that. It's really more like having a serious illness, such as mononucleosis or Lyme disease, only without the infection. In fact, these maladies and others that are accompanied by general malaise in athletes are sometimes misdiagnosed by family doctors as "overtraining." Overtraining is the worst thing that can happen to an athlete, short of a life-threatening illness. The only way to reverse the condition is by complete rest. This could take weeks or even months. Overtraining is not something to be taken lightly.

[Are You Overtrained?]

Overtraining is often described as a chronically decreased capacity for exercise, resulting from an imbalance between stress and rest. But even this is too tame to present the complete picture. If you become overtrained, you can expect a smorgasbord of serious symptoms, ranging from behavioral (such as depression) to physical (such as muscle soreness) (see Table 7.3). Part of the problem in diagnosis is that the symptoms are not the same for every overtrained athlete, or even between different bouts of overtraining in the same athlete.

Note that physical indicators of overtraining include "resting heart rate change" and "lower exercise heart rate." Your heart's pumping rate is the result of the interactions of the sympathetic and parasympathetic nervous systems that make up the autonomic nervous system. As described in Chapter 2, the sympathetic system increases heart rate, while the parasympathetic slows it down. So when you exercise, your nervous systems monitor the demands of the working muscles for oxygen and fuel (and other things) and then regulates how fast your heart beats, in order to keep up with the demand. The same process is used during rest. The autonomic nervous system usually works quite well, but when overtrained it gets a little mixed up and may keep the resting heart rate a bit higher or lower than the demands from the rest of the body require.

In endurance athletes, heart rate tends to be slowed down during the early stages of overtraining, when the sympathetic nervous system is dominant. Note that this is the same thing that happens when your fitness is improving. But if you have brought yourself to a state

BEHAVIORAL SYMPTOMS	PHYSICAL SYMPTOMS
Apathy	Reduced performance
Lethargy	Weight change
Depression	Resting heart rate change
Poor concentration	Muscle soreness and pain
Sleep disturbances	Rapid heart rate after exercise
Irritability	Diarrhea
Decreased libido (sex drive)	Elevated basal metabolic rate
Clumsiness	Upper respiratory infection
Increased thirst	Changes in blood pressure
Sluggishness	Lower exercise heart rate
Loss of appetite	Slow-healing cuts
Emotional instability	Easily fatigued

Table 7.3. Behavioral and Physical Symptoms of Overtraining

of overtraining by doing too much high-intensity training, your parasympathetic system may be working overtime, thus speeding up your resting heart rate.

Some of the symptoms mentioned in Table 7.1 can be classified by the nervous system with which they are associated. For example, sympathetic overtraining can be identified by the following:

• Increased resting heart rate
• Increased blood pressure
• Loss of appetite
• Decreased body weight
• Sleep disturbances
• Emotional instability and irritability
• Elevated basal metabolic rate (you burn more calories during the day)

Signs of parasympathetic overtraining include the following:

• Rapid recovery of heart rate after exercise
• Decreased resting heart rate
• Low exercise heart rate
• Good appetite
• Lethargy
• Depression
• Low lactate levels during exercise
• Easily fatigued
• Decreased resting blood pressure

Of the two types, sympathetic overtraining seems to be the type most commonly identified in the research, but that may be because this type is found mostly in young athletes who make up the bulk of the subjects in scientific studies. Older athletes, who are seldom studied,

REST

TESTS FOR OVERTRAINING

Heart rate, taken first thing in the morning when you wake up, by itself is not a good indicator of whether you are overtrained. Something called the *orthostatic* test, however, has been shown in some research to be a better predictor. Here's how it works.

Wearing a heart rate monitor, lie down for 10 minutes. Check your heart rate and then stand up. At 15 seconds after standing, check your heart rate again. Look at your heart rate again at 2 minutes. The 15-second, peak heart rate is usually interpreted to reflect parasympathetic nervous activity and the 2-minute heart rate sympathetic activity. They *both* are good indicators of overtraining. Some studies have shown that the standing heart rate at 2 minutes is elevated when overtrained. One study of Finnish athletes showed a 10-beat-per-minute increase at 2 minutes in overtrained athletes.

Another alternative that also may be better than checking morning heart rate when you awake is sleeping heart rate average. Two studies showed it to be a more reliable predictor of your rest-stress status. Simply wear a heart rate monitor while sleeping and record the average for the night in a daily log. Look for any unusual increases or decreases in average heart rate over several days. One study, using well-trained, young cyclists as subjects, found a 10 percent increase in sleeping heart rate average when overtrained. This self-test may prove a bit uncomfortable, but is done by some athletes who are training at a high workload and want to make sure they avoid overtraining.

---

are probably more likely to show signs of parasympathetic training.

Some studies have also shown that when an athlete is overtrained, heart rate during exercise is lower compared with when not overtrained. But other studies have shown no difference for exercising heart rate, whether overtrained or well-rested. Of course, when an athlete is in good shape the exercise heart rate will come down for any given level of exercise intensity. This confuses things even more. So, once again, we are left somewhat in the dark when it comes to heart rates telling us whether we need more rest or not. See the "Rest" sidebar above for ways to test whether or not you're overtraining.

The smart athlete understands that when they start to feel invincible, disaster is just one training mistake away. One bad decision made at the precipice of overtraining, such as doing a few more intervals or going a few more miles, and it's all over. Highly motivated, emotionally driven, young, or novice athletes are far less likely to realize when they are doing too much than is a seasoned veteran. That's yet another reason why most athletes are better off training under the guidance of a coach.

So if it's difficult to recognize overtraining, how do you avoid it and still train hard enough to achieve your goals? Several markers may predict when you are exceeding your overtraining threshold and need to be cautious:

- Fatigue that doesn't go away despite 48 hours of active recovery. Your legs feel tired or you feel a general bodily weariness that lingers even after you've taken it easy for 2 days.

- The loss of control of emotions—evidence of anger, feeling sorry for yourself, moodiness, depression, grumpiness. In short, you're hard to live with. Your spouse or roommate may be the first to recognize this.

- Self-confidence is diminished. This may be the best marker, but it's hard to assess. One way to do it may be found in trying to visualize accomplishing a high goal. If it seems out of reach and farfetched, self-confidence may be low and you may be overtraining.

- Fitness declines. The most obvious marker that appears in the overtrained athlete is a drop in performance. Even though the training workload is getting harder, once a state of overtraining is reached the capacity to go fast or do a long workout or event declines. Fitness is being lost despite increases in the frequency, intensity, or duration of workouts. This is illustrated in Figure 7.1.

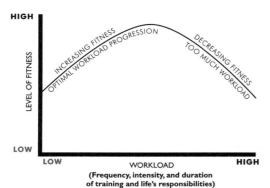

Fig. 7.1. The overtraining curve

When any of these markers show up and linger for more than 2 or 3 days, there's a good chance that your overtraining threshold has been exceeded. At this point the workload, especially the intensity of training, must be reduced or all training stopped immediately until you are back to normal. In the early stages, this could take 3 to 5 days. While taking a break from working out, evaluate how you did this to yourself and what adjustments are needed as you start back.

[Preventing Overtraining]

The best way to prevent overtraining is the liberal use of rest. Just as every week should include at least as many easy days as hard, you should have easy weeks and even easy months. If you make a mistake in training, make it on the side of too much easy training. It is far better to be undertrained and eager than overtrained and apathetic.

Of course, overtraining doesn't result just from exercising too much. You could be "overliving." A 50-hour-per-week job, two kids to raise, a house and yard to maintain, and other responsibilities all take their toll psychologically if not also physically. As an amateur athlete, training just happens to be the one thing you can control. It's doubtful that you would call the boss to ask for a day off since you're not racing well.

OVERLOAD TRAINING FOR GREATER FITNESS

Chronic exercise produces greater fitness through a process known as *adaptation*. Regular, consistent, intensity-appropriate workouts result in the ability to do more exercise as the body grows stronger. As adaptation occurs, marked by improving performance, the amount of high-intensity heart rate training can eventually be increased. So the workload must rise if fitness improvement is to continue. You probably already recognize this phenomenon and allow for it by gradually increasing the number of intervals within workouts, extending the length of workouts, or doing work intervals at a higher heart rate or greater speed.

This is a normal way to train and, given enough weeks of training, produces excellent fitness. It is possible, however, to increase the rate at which fitness improves by briefly flirting with your overtraining threshold.

[Overtraining Threshold]

The workload at which overtraining first appears—the overtraining threshold—is a moving target. The number of days of hard training that result in overtraining when fitness is low early in the year may be easily tolerated when fitness is high later in the season. A considerable amount of research and athlete experience has shown that when one trains at a level that would produce overtraining if continued long enough, but then stops after a few days to recover for several days, fitness will soon soar after the rest cycle. This is called *overload training*.

Overload training usually involves increasing the amount of time in Zones 3, 4, 5a, 5b, and 5c for a week or two, followed by a few days of combined passive and active recovery. The key to making this work *for* you instead of *against* you is to stop the high-intensity workouts short of the overtraining threshold, which is generally in the neighborhood of 2 to 3 weeks, and begin a period of rest. Since you never know exactly where that threshold is, it's best to be a bit conservative

when deciding on the number of days of intense workouts, while at the same time carefully monitoring your body to detect signs that you may be doing too much high-intensity or going too long before recovering. Table 7.4 provides an example of normal and overload training.

The overload period is 10 days of increased intensity followed by 5 days of rest and recovery.

[Supercompensation]

It appears that exceeding the overtraining threshold for a few days stimulates the body to *supercompensate*, becoming significantly more fit than when training was conducted with more moderate amounts of higher intensity training and frequent rest. This is very risky and must be done with great caution. You could easily wind up overtrained and ruin an entire season. The key to this form of training is to keep the overload period brief and to follow it immediately with lots of rest and recovery time.

Younger, experienced, and highly fit athletes *may* be able to handle 10 to 14 days of intense overload workouts. Older athletes should stay well below this range. The number of recovery days varies with individuals and could be as brief as half the number of days spent overtraining or as long as the number of overtraining days. For example, if you did 10 days of overload training, you would probably need between 5 and 10 days of rest and recovery. The first time you try overload training, start with a small number of hard days followed by a large number of recovery days, just to be on the safe side. It's during the recovery period that the body will adapt and become more fit than if training had been at a moderate, normal level of training—unless you did too much. If you did,

DAY	NORMAL	WORKOUT MAX HR ZONE	OVERLOAD	MAX HR ZONE
Monday	Strength work	N/A	Strength work	N/A
Tuesday	Cruise intervals	5a	Cruise intervals	5a
Wednesday	Recovery	1	Tempo intervals	3
Thursday	Aerobic capacity intervals	5b	Aerobic capacity intervals	5b
Friday	Recovery	1	Steady tempo	3
Saturday	Steady tempo	3	30-30s	5b
Sunday	Low AeT, overdistance	2	High AeT	2
Monday	Strength work	N/A	Strength work	N/A
Tuesday	Cruise intervals	5a	Cruise intervals	5a
Wednesday	Recovery	1	Tempo intervals	3
Thursday	Aerobic capacity intervals	5b	Recovery	1
Friday	Recovery	1	Recovery	1
Saturday	Steady tempo	3	Recovery	1
Sunday	Low AeT, overdistance	2	Recovery	1
Monday	Strength work	N/A	Recovery	1

Table 7.4. A Comparison of 15 Days of Normal and Overload Training for a Young, Fit Athlete in the Build Period of the Training Season

then you are simply overtrained and the season is over. *Be cautious!*

Overload training should not be done more often than about once every 8 weeks or so. To do it more often is to also risk overtraining. Such an exercise program, including the extended recovery period, should end at least 3 weeks before an important event, so that you can make sure you are fully rested before starting to peak.

TRIMP

Earlier, this chapter introduced the idea that fitness results from stress being applied to the body, followed by adequate rest (the formula is fitness = stress − rest). The trick is to gradually increase the stress and always provide for adequate rest. So how do you know how much stress is being applied through workouts? Knowing workout duration is not enough. Saying you worked out for an hour doesn't tell us anything about how hard the workout was. In the same way, knowing intensity is not enough, because that doesn't address how long the intense portions of the workout lasted. Obviously, we need some combination of duration and intensity to know how much stress a given workout produces.

In 1975 Eric Banister of the University of Victoria in British Columbia, Canada, introduced the concept of TRaining IMPulse (Trimp). This is a simple way of using a heart rate monitor to calculate stress from a workout and also the accumulated stress of several workouts during a week. It is defined as:

Trimp = training duration x training intensity

There are two Trimp methods that may be used to estimate stress in your workouts—Basic and Advanced.

[Basic Trimp]

This method works best for the general fitness enthusiast as well as for the person new to sport whose workouts are rather simple—usually steady state, as in exercising continuously for 30 minutes within a narrow heart rate range. Basic Trimp is very easy to use. All you need to know from your heart rate monitor is how many minutes the workout lasted and what your average heart rate was. Multiply these two numbers and you have a Basic Trimp stress load for that workout. For example, let's say you exercised for 30 minutes at an average heart rate of 132. Your Trimp for that workout would be found by multiplying these two numbers:

Trimp = 30 minutes x 132 average heart rate
= 3,960

In keeping with the idea that you want to alternate hard and easy days throughout the week to provide for recovery from stress, and using Basic Trimp to "score" the workouts, a week of exercise may look something like the example in Table 7.5.

In this example you can see that the athlete has alternated low-Trimp days (Monday, Tues-

DAY	DURATION	AVERAGE HR	TRIMP
Mon	Day off	N/A	0
Tues	30 min	132	3,960
Wed	45 min	145	6,525
Thurs	20 min	128	2,560
Fri	35 min	155	5,425
Sat	30 min	130	3,900
Sun	60 min	131	7,860

Table 7.5. Example of Basic Trimp Method Used to Manage the Stress of Harder and Easier Training for One Week

day, Thursday, and Saturday) and high-Trimp days (Wednesday, Friday, and Sunday). Notice also in the example for Sunday that while the average heart rate was low (131) the Trimp was relatively high (7,860), because of the long duration of the workout. Another hard training day on Friday (5,425) was accomplished by doing just the opposite—combining high intensity with low duration. Either way, the stress is high on those days, meaning the body needs rest fairly soon—usually the next day.

The beauty of this is that you can plan a week using Trimp as a guide. All you need to do is determine what the duration and approximate heart rate intensity will be. You can then schedule easy-rest (low-Trimp) and hard-stress (high-Trimp) days on a calendar or in your training diary. That way you'll ensure that you balance rest with stress (so long as you stick with your plan!).

The weakness of the Basic Trimp method is that it does not account for a variety of intensities that last for varying amounts of time in a workout, such as when doing intervals. During the work interval portions of a session, the average heart rate may be 170, but only 130 during the recovery intervals. The average of these could be in the neighborhood of 150 or probably much less for the entire workout once warm-up and cool-down times and intensities are factored in. The average heart rate could wind up being in the low 140s. And yet the workout was obviously hard, owing to the high-heart rate intervals. That's where *Advanced* Trimp comes in handy.

[Advanced Trimp]

This method varies from Basic Trimp by using time in each heart rate zone, instead of average heart rate for the total workout, to determine how stressful the workout is. So by doing it this way, high- and low-intensity exercise is not diluted by averaging. And yet this method is still easy to use. All you do is multiply the number of minutes in each heart rate zone by the zone's numeric name. So, for example, 10 minutes in Zone 2 would count as 20 Trimp "points" ($10 \times 2 = 20$). Of course, for this to work you need a heart rate monitor that keeps track of time in each of the five zones. These devices are usually a bit more expensive than those that simply report all exercise time as a single number, but it is money well spent if you are serious about your training.

Using Advanced Trimp, a 1-hour, Aerobic Capacity interval workout made up of 5, 3-minute work intervals with 3-minute recoveries, a 20-minute warm-up, and a 10-minute cool down might be "scored" like Table 7.6.

Notice that Zone 5 is not subdivided into 5a, 5b, and 5c. One reason for this is that heart rate monitors don't allow for seven zones. And, besides that obvious reason, another is that heart rate monitors are not very good at meas-

uring Zone 5c, since time in this zone is of necessity brief and heart rate seldom has enough time to "catch up" with how hard you are going before it begins dropping.

Also notice that in this example even though the athlete was doing 15 minutes at Zone 5b intensity, the total Zone 5 time is only 11 minutes. That's because, once again, heart rate responds slowly to the body's demands because of high intensity on the first few work intervals. By the way, don't let this heart rate lag cause you to decide that the work interval doesn't really start until heart rate reaches the target level. There is no point to doing that. When performing intervals you are attempting to improve the fitness of far more systems than simply the cardiovascular. The timing of the interval starts as soon as the high-intensity output (pace or power) begins, not when heart rate achieves the targeted zone.

The score using the Advanced Trimp method is always going to be far different than that found when using Basic Trimp, so it's not possible to blend the two. You must use either one or the other to remain consistent and collect data that is meaningful.

HR ZONE	MINUTES IN ZONE	TRIMP POINTS
1	19	19
2	17	34
3	7	21
4	6	24
5	11	55
Total Trimp Score for the Workout		153

Table 7.6. Example of Advanced Trimp Used to Score a Workout

Advanced Trimp is a great way to keep track of the stress your training creates, in order to balance it with an appropriate amount of rest. Table 7.7 illustrates how a week of training might look for an athlete who uses Advanced Trimp to balances stress and rest.

Sometimes it's helpful to see concepts such as this in graph form. Figure 7.2 shows how the above week looks in a bar graph:

In the graphic display of the example used here, you can easily see the balancing of hard days and easy days with the stress being applied on Tuesday, Thursday, Saturday, and Sunday. Since Saturday and Sunday are such hard days back to back, our wise athlete is taking Monday off from exercise altogether.

In the same manner we can view a longer period of time such as 8 weeks to see how stress and rest are balanced for the athlete in our example, as shown in Figure 7.3.

You can see by this example of 8 weeks of accumulated weekly Trimp scores that the ath-

lete has provided for increasing amounts of stress weekly, as adaptation was occurring, and also allowed for recovery every 4 weeks by scheduling easier training in weeks 4 and 8. Note that none of these examples is supposed to show precisely how many Trimp points you should aim for in a given workout or week. These are merely examples to show one way that training stress may be distributed, as measured by your heart rate monitor. You can schedule hard and easy exercise days in a variety of ways, which Chapter 8 discusses in greater detail.

[Trimp and Triathlon]

Be aware that neither Basic or Advanced Trimp works very well for triathletes. The reason for this is that a bike ride may go on for several hours, far longer than a typical run would last. And the longest runs are always longer than the longest swims when training for any triathlon event. Since every minute of workout time counts toward Trimp points, the bike workouts

DAY	WORKOUT	WORKOUT DURATION (min.)	TIME BY ZONE	TRIMP SCORE
Monday	Day off	0	–	0
Tuesday	Aerobic Capacity Intervals	60	1–19, 2–17, 3–7, 4–6, 5–11	153
Wednesday	Recovery	45	1–45, 2–0, 3–0, 4–0, 5–0	45
Thursday	Cruise Steady State	60	1–15, 2–12, 3–3, 4–30, 5–0	168
Friday	Recovery	45	1–45, 2–0, 3–0, 4–0, 5–0	45
Saturday	Cruise Intervals	70	1–12, 2–8, 3–6, 4–41, 5–3	225
Sunday	Low AeT	120	1–30, 2–90, 3–0, 4–0, 5–0	210
Total Trimp Score for the Workout				846

Table 7.7. Example of One Week of Training Scored Using the Advanced Trimp Method

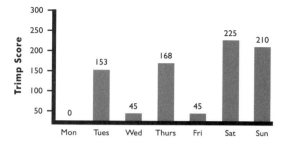

Fig. 7.2. Graphic display of an example of Advanced Trimp weekly scoring to show how stress varies from day to day

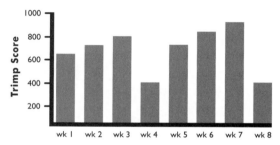

Fig. 7.3. Graphic display of eight weeks of Advanced Trimp weekly scoring showing a balancing of hard and easy weeks of training

will usually represent a far greater portion of the weekly score. The swim will typically represent a much smaller portion of the time and Trimp points for the triathlete. In other words, 5 minutes of Zone 1 on the bike scores the same as 1 minute of Zone 5 running or swimming. And there can be a lot of Zone 1 time spent on the bike in a week.

So long as the amounts of swim, bike, and run training time remain much the same from week to week, there is no problem. But the first time the triathlete reduces bike time for a week while emphasizing the run or, especially, the swim, it is highly likely that the weekly score would indicate a low-stress week even though hard run or swim training may have been included instead of long, easy bike rides. It may be possible to correct for this by dividing Trimp scores for a run workout by 2 and all bike

workouts by 4. This is by no means a perfect way of resolving this issue, but can provide some level of reliability if used consistently.

In the same way, Trimp does not work very well for speed skill work or for nonaerobic, cross training activities such as weight training or other strength or power-development exercises.

THE **HEART** OF THE MATTER

In this chapter you learned about the importance of balancing stress and rest. The known causes of fatigue and how to manage each of them in order to train for greater fitness and higher performance were introduced. We examined how the repeated experience and long duration of fatigue without allowing for rest leads to overtraining. Whether or not an athlete becomes overtrained depends on how high (or low) the athlete's overtraining threshold is. This threshold is determined both by the intensity and duration of training sessions and by how many consecutive or nearly consecutive days the threshold is exceeded. It rises as fitness improves. Exceeding it for short periods with overload training actually creates high fitness through an adaptive process called supercompensation. A simple and effective way to monitor and regulate adaptation, whether from normal or overload training, involves using a heart rate monitor to keep track of the Training Impulse—Trimp.

Chapter 8 pulls together many of the loose ends we have created in the last five chapters by showing you how to plan using a successful, long-term approach to training.

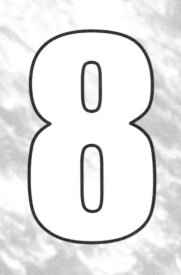

8

PERIODIZATION AND PEAK FITNESS

Training is largely an act of faith. Athletes have faith that the workouts they do will result in greater fitness in time for their targeted events. They have faith that the stress created by a workout and by the subsequent rest is adequate to produce a positive adaptation. They have faith that they aren't overtraining or undertraining. It's no wonder that athletes often lack confidence in their preparation and question if it's working.

Using a heart rate monitor removes a lot of this guesswork. It enables you to measure and distribute the training load effectively, and with some degree of certainty. You can gauge fitness progress by conducting periodic field tests or by comparing your workout heart rates with pace or power, as described in Chapter 4. With a heart rate monitor you can create the sort of training variety that the body thrives on, as shown in Chapters 5 and 6. Balancing stress with rest can be accomplished with the Trimp method, described in Chapter 7. Your heart rate monitor is a powerful tool that helps you to train with much more confidence—*if* you know how to use it.

How you arrange workouts also has a lot to do with your confidence. A proven method for doing this is something called *periodization*. This is simply a way of organizing training by dividing the season into periods of time, each period having a unique purpose. As the season progresses, these periods change the stresses applied to the body. Basically, workouts become more challenging and begin to take on the characteristics of your next high-priority event. As the intensity and duration of workouts become more difficult just before your targeted event, you are essentially doing mini-races as workouts separated by easy, recovery days.

Then in the last few days before the competition, rest is really emphasized with just enough intensity to maintain fitness.

The final week before the race can be a mentally trying time. You are likely to have uncertainty about race readiness, and that's when serious self-doubt begins to set in. It's not unusual for athletes to try to "prove" to themselves that they are ready by doing too much hard training the week of the event. This usually has the opposite effect and leaves them tired on race day, when being rested is critical.

This chapter deals with that dynamic, describing how to go about tapering and peaking for an event while reducing self-doubt by using the same strategy I use with the athletes whom I coach. Peaking is the process of becoming race ready just in time for the race. Tapering simply means that the training load is being reduced in the final weeks before the competition. To understand tapering and peaking, you must first be familiar with periodization.

PERIODIZATION OF HEART RATE

Periodization was first described early in the twentieth century by Russian sport scientists and refined over the next hundred years by scientists, coaches, and athletes in all sports. In the 1970s endurance athletes in the West began to study and use the concepts of periodization that made the Eastern Bloc countries, especially the Soviet Union and East Germany, practically unbeatable in Olympic medal count competition. Today periodization is used by nearly all world-class competitors and most serious amateur athletes as well.

There are other ways of organizing the season besides periodization, but this system has become such a dominant force in sport that many now think of it as a "principle of training," which it definitely is not. Other systems for organizing training, while not as popular and thor-

oughly studied as periodization, can also be effective. However, I encourage you to use periodization, since it has been proven to produce outstanding fitness regardless of the athlete's experience, training capacity, or level of competition.

[The Periods]

In the classic periodization model, the season is divided into long, medium, and short periods, hence the name "periodization." The longest periods, called "macrocycles," usually last for several months and end with an A-priority event that is one of the most important competitions of the season (race priorities are described in "Step 6" of Chapter 9). Typically, two or three macrocycles occur during an athlete's year.

The shortest periods are called "microcycles" and are made up of a few consecutive days of training sessions. Microcycles are usually one week long, but can be of any such brief duration. For most athletes, 7 days works best, since their lives already revolve around a schedule of activities that happen in 7-day cycles. Trying to fit a 10-day microcycle, or some other length, into a 7-day lifestyle makes training quite a challenge.

Between the long macrocycles and the short microcycles are the medium-length peri-

MACROCYCLE	TRAINING YEAR					
	PREPARATION			COMPETITION		TRANSITION
MESOCYCLES	GENERAL PREP		SPECIFIC PREP	PRE-COMP	COMPETITION	TRANSITION
	PREP	BASE	BUILD	PEAK	RACE	TRANSITION
MICROCYCLES	1 / 2	3 / 4 / 5 / 6 / 7 / 8	/ / / / / / WEEKS 9–42 / / / / / /	43 / 44 / 45 / 46 / 47 / 48 / 49 / 50 / 51 / 52		

Fig. 8.1. Periodization terminology

PERIOD	LENGTH (WEEKS)	PURPOSE	PRIMARY ABILITIES*	SECONDARY ABILITIES*
Prep	2–6	Begin training to train, general fitness (cross-training)	E	F
Base	6–12	Develop basic abilities, introduce ME, increase training volume, general fitness (sport-specific)	E,F,SS	ME
Build	3–9	Develop advanced abilities, race-specific fitness, increase race-like intensity, slightly reduce volume, maintain basic abilities	ME,AE,P	E,F,SS
Peak	1–2	Simulate portions of race, reduce volume significantly, increase rest, maintain fitness	ME,AE,P	E
Race	1–2	Maintain race intensity, emphasize rest, focus on race	ME,AE,P	E
Transition	1–4	Recover, rest, rejuvenate	E	—

* E = endurance, F = force, SS = speed skill, ME = muscular endurance,
AE = anaerobic endurance, P = power (see Chapter 6 for an explanation of the abilities)

Table 8.1. Mesocycle Descriptions

ods, called "mesocycles." These are groupings of microcycles that have a similar purpose. It is common to give mesocycles names, since they are referred to so frequently in the training process. Figure 8.1 lists many of the names often used for mesocycles by sport scientists, coaches, and athletes. The names that we will use here, in their order of occurrence in the season, are Prep, Base, Build, Peak, Race, and Transition.

[Period Purpose]

As mentioned, each mesocycle has a training purpose. These purposes are related to the Training Triad abilities illustrated in Figure 6.1. Table 8.1 lists the mesocycles, along with their durations, purposes, and emphasis on both primary and secondary abilities. A primary ability is

one on which most of your microcycle workouts focus. They are the primary emphasis of your training at a given point in time. Secondary abilities are those you've included for the first time in a macrocycle or those that you previously developed and you're now simply trying to maintain.

Let's look at maintenance of fitness, since this is such an important key to periodization and is usually messed up by athletes. Examples of ability maintenance in the above table are endurance, force, and speed skill during the Build period.

To maintain an ability, you only need do it about half as frequently as when you were first developing the ability. For example, to develop a high level of endurance in the Base period you may do a long-duration AeT workout (Zone 2) once each week. But by the time you are in the Build period and this ability is well established, all that is needed to maintain endurance is a long AeT workout every other week—half as frequently. That frees some of your time in the Build period to concentrate on the primary, more race-specific abilities of muscular endurance, anaerobic endurance, or power (Chapter 9 will help you determine which abilities to concentrate on, to suit your unique needs). An abil-

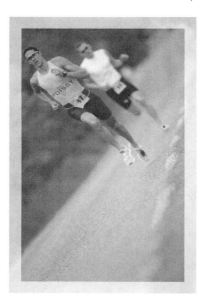

ity can usually be maintained in this manner for the final 12 weeks necessary to specifically prepare for an A-priority race. Individual limits, of course, govern how long an athlete can maintain an ability in this manner. The better established that the ability is initially, the longer that it will hold up with a reduced frequency of training. This is one reason why the Base mesocycle period is so important. When done right the Base period establishes high levels of fitness for the most basic abilities—endurance, force, and speed skill—which then are easily maintained in the Build period.

The best reason for using periodization in your training is that it *works*. A properly designed and followed plan using the concepts described here, and further explained in Chapter 9, will bring you to a peak of fitness at the times when your most important events are scheduled. I've seen it happen repeatedly with athletes at all levels of performance. Most who follow such a program for the first time are amazed at the way they feel on race day, and their excellent results confirm the benefits of such planning and organization.

PEAKING **AND HEART RATE**

An issue that many athletes find mysterious is how to come into competitive "form" at the times in the season when their most important events are scheduled. Form is a vague concept used by athletes in some sports to describe when they are ready to compete. The word has its roots in eighteenth-century horse racing when sheets, or printed "forms," would be provided for race track bettors showing the past performances of each horse.

Exercise scientist Andrew Coggan, Ph.D., defines form as the timely combination of fitness and freshness. Fitness has to do with how well the body's many systems function at a given point in time. A fit endurance athlete has optimized the cardiovascular, metabolic, respiratory, muscular, and nervous systems. A fresh athlete is one who is rested in all systems and ready to go. It's possible to be fit but not fresh, as a result of lots of heavy training but not much resting leading into an event. You're tired. It's also possible to be fresh but not fit. You've been taking it easy for too long and are undertrained. Bringing fitness and freshness together at the same time is called "peaking" and is the underlying purpose of training for the competitive athlete in the last few days and weeks before a race.

To increase freshness as you get closer in time to the competition, you cut back on the training workload by reducing the duration and frequency of workouts. You include more easy, recovery workouts or days off each week. As a result you become more fresh. To maintain the fitness created over the previous weeks and months of training, you do a few key workouts at race intensity and otherwise train easily between them. Getting the intensity of your workouts just right is why your heart rate monitor is so critical to peaking.

[How Peaking Works]

Actually, sports scientists don't fully understand the physiology of why tapering the training load, by increasing the amount of rest over a few days or weeks before a race, results in increased fitness. But they *do* know of several changes that occur in the body with such training. The most notable is an increase in strength and power. Others are reduced blood acidity, increased blood volume, greater red blood cell concentration for oxygen transport, increased carbohydrate storage in the muscles, and even sharper mental skills.

Although tapering the training load before important competitions is widely practiced by top athletes, many are afraid that cutting back on training will cause a loss of fitness. They are wrong. Numerous research studies support and confirm the wisdom of reduced training. Several that used athletes from many sports found that reducing training by more than half of what was normal for two to three weeks produced no losses of fitness or performance. Others have shown improvements in performance when the tapering off was done in a certain way.

In a classic study conducted at the University of Illinois a group of runners and cyclists who greatly cut back on their training, by reducing the frequency and duration of workouts while keeping their intensities the same, significantly improved both their aerobic capacities, an important measure of fitness, and their endurance performance. Those who reduced intensity but kept frequency and duration the same lost fitness. All the evidence is in, then: Do *not* decrease the intensity of training as you approach your most important races.

Take special note here of the ingredients for a successful taper, according to this and similar research studies—reduced weekly volume (freshness) and an emphasis on intensity (fitness). So the key to tapering is keeping workout intensity—heart rate—at high levels while resting more. Again, here's where your heart rate monitor is essential to your success.

The tapering of duration and frequency occurs during the final two periods before the competition—the Peak and Race mesocycles.

[The Peak Mesocycle]

The Peak mesocycle typically begins about two or three weeks before the competition. The length of this mesocycle varies by sport, fitness level, and nature of the targeted event. Sports that are orthopedically stressful, such as running, require a long period of tapering. Reducing frequency and duration, starting three weeks or even more before an important competition, is common for runners. A sport such as swimming that has no hard surface pounding associated with it can benefit from a shorter taper period. For swimmers, 7 to 14 days of tapering is common. Other sports, such as rowing and cycling, will fall between these two extremes. A triathlete will taper each of the three sports at different rates.

The greater your fitness is, the longer the taper should be. Another way of looking at this is that if your fitness is poor, perhaps because you got started late in preparing for your event, you need all the time you can get to build fitness. So in this situation the Peak period is shortened in favor of a longer Build period. The taper may only be for 10 days.

The longer the event is that you are training for, the longer the taper should last. For example, a runner may taper for 3 weeks for a marathon but only taper 10 days for a 5k race. Longer races usually mean greater training loads, with an emphasis on long-duration workouts. Long workouts take a greater toll on the body than short workouts, and so more time is necessary to recover and rebuild reserves.

During the Peak mesocycle, reduce training volume by 20 to 30 percent every 3 to 4 days. The shorter the taper length is, the greater the reduction should be. Again, do not decrease the intensity or heart rates of your workouts, only their duration.

The frequency of your workouts, or how often you train, may also be slightly decreased while tapering so long as you have been doing at least 5 or 6 workouts in a sport in a normal week during the preceding Build mesocycle. A triathlete, for example, who has been doing 3 swims, 3 bike rides, and 3 runs weekly should not decrease the frequency of these sessions, as it is already marginal. When the frequency of training gets too low, you may experience a loss of economy—how efficiently you move. Essentially, your movements may become sloppy as the muscles forget how to move economically. Swimmers call this losing their "feel" for the water.

The basis of the training structure for the Peak period is to simulate the intensity of a portion of the targeted race every third or fourth day until 7 days before the event. To do a simulation workout, you select a segment of the event that is critical to your success and practice exactly how you will gauge heart rate and effort for that segment. For example, there may be a hill on the course that is critical to how well you perform on the day. Find a similar hill, warm up, and then simulate the intensity you plan to use in the race. Or it may be that the course is flat and you need to maintain a specific intensity to reach your goal. Rehearse that intensity in each of the simulation workouts. That intensity could be based on heart rate—or on pace, power, or perceived exertion as compared with heart rate.

Whatever you decide is the portion of the race that is critical, make the simulation a dress rehearsal in as many ways as possible. This may involve clothing, equipment, mental approach, refueling, or anything else that is a part of your race-day strategy. One or two of the simulation workouts in the Peak period may be a C-priority race, done as a tune-up.

Note that while the intensity of your simulation is critical to the success of your Peak period, going beyond the targeted race intensity is not beneficial and may even be counterproductive. For example, a marathoner who sets a goal of running a 7-minute pace in Zone 3 should do simulations only at this intensity—not a 6-minute pace in Zone 5.

So if you do a race simulation every three or four days in the Peak period, what is done in the 2 or 3 days between these workouts? You do short, easy, recovery workouts or you take a

DAY	DURATION (MIN)	WORKOUT TYPE
Mon	0	Day off
Tues	45	Short and easy
Wed	90	Simulation
Thurs	45	Short and easy
Fri	45	Short and easy
Sat	70	Simulation
Sun	40	Short and easy
Mon	0	Day off
Tues	55	Simulation
Wed	35	Short and easy
Thurs	35	Short and easy
Fri	45	Simulation
Sat	30	Short and easy
Sun	30	Short and easy

Table 8.2. Example of a Two-Week Peak Period

day off. The idea is to be fully recovered and ready to go again for the next simulation. Table 8.2 offers an example of a two-week Peak period.

[The Race Mesocycle]

The week of the goal competition is called the Race mesocycle. While generally one week, it could include two or three weeks of back-to-back, A-priority races. However, it becomes increasingly difficult to maintain race fitness with reduced training over several weeks. With a two-week Peak period of ever-decreasing workout durations, as illustrated in Table 8.2, each additional week of low-duration workouts gradually results in a loss of endurance. With enough such low-volume weeks, you would eventually

be unfit for long-endurance events. If it is the end of the season and you have only two or three important races remaining on the schedule, this is not a problem. But a long taper earlier in the season means that you must go back to Base period training to rebuild endurance and possibly other abilities. And the longer your taper was, the more time it will take to reestablish fitness. So be quite cautious with how long you stay in the Race period. An overly long taper may well mean that your fitness won't be what it should for subsequent high-priority races later in the season.

The underlying theme of the Race period is the same as for the Peak period—rehearse race intensity while resting. The greatest difference now is that the workouts are even more brief and the simulations are composed of short work intervals with long recoveries. The work intervals are about 90 seconds in duration and done at the highest intensity planned for the goal event. The recoveries are twice as long as the work intervals, so about 3 minutes. These intervals are done several times throughout the week but decrease by one interval each day as the week progresses, with the greatest number being 5 or 6 early in the week. Table 8.3 illustrates a Race week using this strategy.

Several research studies have shown this strategy of decreasing racelike intervals to be effective in boosting fitness in the last few days before a competition. In one such study conducted by Shepley and colleagues at McMaster University in Ontario, Canada, a group of competitive college cross-country runners improved their endurance at a one-mile pace by 22 percent in just one week following a program similar to the one shown in Table 8.3. They ran 330 meters farther at their best 1500-

DAYS UNTIL RACE	WORKOUT
6	Warm-up, 6 racelike intervals, cool-down
5	Warm-up, 5 racelike intervals, cool-down
4	Warm-up, 4 racelike intervals, cool-down
3	Warm-up, 3 racelike intervals, cool-down
2	Day off
1	Warm-up, 1 racelike interval, cool-down
Race	—

Table 8.3. Example of Race Period Workouts

meter pace, following a similar training pattern for one week. The runners in the study who reduced volume by the same amount as the first group but ran with a slow pace improved only 6 percent, running 90 meters farther. A third group that took the entire week off to rest unfortunately experienced a decline in performance of 3 percent covering 45 meters less at their best 1500-meter pace.

Notice in Table 8.3 that two days before the race is a day off from training. It's generally a good idea to get one day of complete rest at some point close to race day. Resting the day before the race is not as effective. Athletes often report that they feel "flat" on race day when doing this. Taking a day off two days before also works out well, because this is a common day for travel to distant events. Being at the race venue the day before also gives you the opportunity to do the last race-like interval workout on a portion of the actual course.

Besides rehearsing race intensity with short intervals each day this week, be sure to allow for plenty of time off for your legs to rest. Don't stand if you can sit. Don't sit if you can lie down. Rest.

THE HEART OF THE MATTER

Periodization is a training strategy that divides the season into periods, each of which has a purpose. Heart rate and other measures of intensity, such as pace and power, gradually take on the qualities of the race as the season progresses. In the final few weeks before an important event, tapering of training volume is introduced. Tapering your workout duration and frequency in the last two to three weeks before an important competition is one aspect of becoming race ready. The other part is keeping your workout intensity high relative to the event for which you are training. The Peak period that initiates this taper lasts one to two weeks and is composed of racelike workout simulations every three to four days with days of rest and recovery between them. In the Race period, the week of the important race, brief interval workouts that get shorter each day are done almost daily. This process has been shown to produce high levels of form—or fitness and freshness—on race day.

9

THE TOTAL HEART RATE TRAINING PROGRAM

This chapter ties together many loose ends, guiding you through the process of developing a detailed heart rate–based training program. By following along with the worksheets in the appendices you'll do exactly what I would do if I was coaching you. I've used the 12-step process described here to prepare athletes for the Olympics, world competitions, and national championships. I've also used it to get novices ready for their first competitions. It works.

You may decide not to complete the worksheets that accompany this chapter, because doing so requires a lot of thinking and soul searching. For athletes who do not have challenging goals, that is understandable. But if you have high athletic aspirations, and especially if there is a sizable gap between your current capability and what is demanded by your goals, then following the step-by-step process in this chapter will greatly increase your chances of success. No one can guarantee your success, however. It will still come down to how dedicated you are to training. That's one of the reasons we all enjoy endurance sport so much—there's no one else to blame or give credit to but us.

The best time in the season to develop your plan using this chapter is at the start of your season, before you do the first workout. But even if you are already into your competitive season as you read this, following along with the worksheets will still give focus to the remainder of your season and help you produce better results. You may find it helpful to return to this chapter before beginning each new season to get organized and give direction to your training.

YOUR TRAINING PLAN

An important key to the success of a training plan based on periodization is the use of your heart rate monitor to closely gauge the intensity of each workout. Intensity has repeatedly been shown by research to be the primary determiner of fitness. Therefore, designing your training plan based on your unique heart rate zones has a lot to do with how well you perform in athletic competition.

Of course, following a plan does not mean doing so rigidly. There will be days when you shouldn't follow the plan because you are not recovered from a previous workout, or you feel a cold coming on, or for whatever reason you sense that the timing is not right to challenge your body. At times like these it is always best to do less—to go short and easy or even take the day off. To do otherwise is to risk illness, injury, burnout, and overtraining. Missing one scheduled workout is preferable to missing one week, or more, of training. Always give yourself permission to do less, and your fitness will bloom and your athletic career will be long and rewarding. If you are ever unsure of what to do—am I catching the flu?—the answer is to do less. "When in doubt leave it out," I tell all the athletes I coach.

Now it's time to tie together much of what you have learned in this book. I will walk you through the steps of designing a seasonal training plan in which heart rate regulates workout intensity. You can use the worksheets in the appendices to help guide you and to record your plan as you follow these steps. By the time you are done with this chapter you will have a total heart rate training plan customized to your unique needs. It will look something like the sample on pages 114–15.

[Step 1: Find Your Lactate Threshold Heart Rate]

Chapter 3 described how to go about finding the single most important heart rate for an endurance athlete—the lactate threshold (LT) heart rate, the heart rate at which you first begin to "redline." Recall that this is used instead of max heart rate to establish training zones, since athletes gauge how intense a workout is by comparing their efforts with the feelings they've experienced when at their LT. This LT heart rate varies fairly widely between athletes who have the same max heart rate.

If you have not already done so, find your unique LT heart rate by going to Appendix 1 and selecting one of the two self-tests described there. Be aware that there is a learning curve associated with all such testing. Athletes invariably start too fast when using the 30-minute time trial method. Be just a bit conservative with how fast you go in the first 10 minutes of this test. and you'll likely finish strongly rather than limping painfully to the finish from having been too eager at the start.

While the graded exercise test prevents you from starting out too fast, it requires having an assistant who can identify ventilatory threshold (VT)—the point at which labored breathing first is heard and you find it quite difficult to talk. That, too, takes some experience, gained from helping you several times on this test. After a few such tests VT becomes rather obvious. But not at first.

It is a good idea to use one of these tests at the end of each mesocycle of training, especially in the last week of the Prep, Base, and Build periods so that heart rate may be adjusted as necessary before going to the next level of training.

If you are a triathlete, you will need to test each sport for LT heart rate, as heart rates vary considerably by sport. But if you have time to test only one right now, assume that your LT heart rate for running is 7 beats higher than for biking, which in turn is 7 beats higher than for swimming. Knowing one LT heart rate and these typical variances will allow you to estimate the other two. For example, if your LT heart rate for biking is 152, by adding 7 you estimate that your run LT heart rate is 159. Subtract 7 and you estimate that your swim LT heart rate is 145. These estimates will do until you have time to run the other two tests.

Record your LT heart rate where requested in Appendix 1.

[Step 2: Determine Your Heart Rate Zones]

Now that your LT heart rate is known, it's time to determine your training zones. Turn to Appendix 2 and find the appropriate table for

Text continued on page 118.

ANNUAL TRAINING PLAN / sample

ATHLETE: Tom Athlete

ANNUAL HOURS: 400

SEASON GOALS:

1. Qualify for Boston Marathon by running 3:20 at Midwest Marathon (most important goal).
2. Run a P.B. of under 40 minutes at Hometown 10k.
3. Finish the Horribly Hilly 30k without walking.

TRAINING OBJECTIVES:

1. Maintain coupling of high Zone 2 heart rate and pace for 2 hours by the end of the Base period.
2. Freebar squat 1.5 x body weight by January 22.
3. Complete a 5k race with an average cadence of 88 by April 23.
4. Take 45 seconds off of my self-test TTT time at heart rate range 141 to 143 by October 1.
5. Complete 15 minutes of Zone 5b intervals at an average pace of under 6 minutes by June 15.

W - Weights
E - Endurance
F - Force
S - Speed Skill
M - Muscular Endurance
A - Anaerobic Endurance
P - Power
T - Weights

WK#	MONDAY	RACES	PRI	PERIOD	HOURS	COMMENTS		W	E	F	S	M	A	P	T
1	Nov 7			Tran	-	Finishing off previous season.	—								
2	Nov 14			"	-	"	—								X
3	Nov 21			Prep	7.0	Start of season.	AA	X	X	X	X				
4	Nov 28			"	7.0		"	X	X	X	X				
5	Dec 5			Base 1	8.0		"	X	X	X	X				
6	Dec 12			"	9.5		MT	X	X	X	X				
7	Dec 19			"	10.5		"	X	X	X	X				
8	Dec 26			"	5.5		MS	X	X	X	X				X
9	Jan 2			Base 2	8.5		"	X	X	X	X	X			
10	Jan 9			"	10.0		"	X	X	X	X	X			
11	Jan 16			"	11.0		"	X	X	X	X	X			
12	Jan 23			"	5.5		SM	X	X		X	X			X
13	Jan 30			Base 3	9.0	Wknd group run—don't race!	"	X	X		X	X			
14	Feb 6			"	10.5	Wknd group run—don't race!	"	X	X		X	X			
15	Feb 13			"	11.5	Wknd group run—don't race!	"	X	X		X	X			
16	Feb 20			"	5.5		"	X	X		X				
17	Feb 27			Build 1	10.0	Start Tuesday track workouts.	"	X	X		X	X	X		
18	Mar 6			"	10.0		"	X	X		X	X	X		
19	Mar 13	Heath Half Marathon	B	"	8.0	Rest for 3 days before race.	"	X	X		X	X	X		
20	Mar 20			"	5.5		"	X	X			X			
21	Mar 27			Build 2	9.5		"	X	X		X	X	X		X

WK#	MONDAY	RACES	PRI	PERIOD	HOURS	COMMENTS	W	E	F	S	M	A	P	T
22	Apr 3			"	9.5		X	X	X	X	X	X		
23	Apr 10			"	9.5		X	X	X	X	X	X		
24	Apr 17	Zucco 5k	C	"	5.5	Concentrate on form & cadence.	X			X				X
25	Apr 24			Peak	8.5				X	X	X			
26	May 1			"	6.5		X			X	X			
27	May 8	Horribly Hilly 30k	A	Race	8.5	Race Sunday. Time includes race.	—		X	X	X	X		
28	May 15			Tran	8.5	3 days of rest.	MT	X	X	X				
29	May 22			Build 1	10.0		"	X	X	X	X	X		
30	May 29			"	10.0		"	X	X	X	X	X		
31	Jun 5			"	10.0		SM	X	X	X	X	X		
32	Jun 12	Post 10k	C	"	5.5	Focus on mile 1 pacing.	"	X						
33	Jun 19			Peak	8.5		"		X	X	X			
34	Jun 26			"	6.5		"		X	X	X			
35	Jul 3	Hometown 10k	A	Race	6.5	Race Sunday. Time includes race.	—		X	X	X	X		
36	Jul 10			Tran	3.0	5 days rest. Start Base 3 on wknd	MT	X	X	X	X	X		
37	Jul 17			Base 3	10.5		MS	X	X	X	X	X		
38	Jul 24			"	11.5		"	X	X	X	X	X		
39	Jul 31			"	5.5	Finish Base 3 on Tues. Then R&R.	"	X	X	X	X	X		X
40	Aug 7			Build 1	10.0	Race refueling!	SM	X	X	X	X	X		
41	Aug 14			"	10.0	"	"	X	X	X	X	X		
42	Aug 21			"	10.0	"	"	X	X	X	X	X		
43	Aug 28	Flat 'n Fast 10k	B	"	5.5	"	"	X	X	X	X			
44	Sep 4			Build 2	9.5	Marathon pacing!	"	X	X	X	X			
45	Sep 11			"	9.5	"	"	X	X	X	X			
46	Sep 18	Zinkgraf 5k	C	"	9.5	Rehearse pre-race meal.	"	X	X	X	X			
47	Sep 25			"	5.5		"	X	X	X	X			
48	Oct 2			Peak	8.5		"		X	X	X			
49	Oct 9			"	6.5		"		X	X	X			
50	Oct 16	Midwest Marathon	A	Race	9.0	Race Sunday. Time includes race.	—		X	X	X			
51	Oct 23			Tran	-		—							
52	Oct 30			"	-		—							

your sport or sports. In the table find your LT heart rate in the bold numbers in the "Zone 5a" column. By reading to the left and right of this LT heart rate across the table, you can see all your training zones. Mark this row so that you may refer to it later. Testing later in the season may modify your LT estimate, necessitating the use of a different row of zones.

[Step 3: Select an Annual Training Plan]

In the following steps you will build a training plan for your season that is unique to your abilities, needs, race schedule, and capacity for training workload. This training plan will serve as a "road map" for your season. You will refer to it often. At the end of each week you will use it to help organize your calendar for the coming week. By scheduling workouts in your appointment calendar, much as you would any other important event, you make sure that training does not get crowded out by the details of life. This training plan will be your guide as you go through the season.

Turn to Appendix 3 where blank Annual Training Plans (ATP) are provided. Here you will find an ATP for single-sport athletes such as runners and cyclists, and also an ATP for triathletes (you may make a copy of the appropriate page). Or go online to www.TargetHRT.com and select "Free Resources." Then save or print the appropriate ATP according to your sport. If you save it to your computer you can do all the following in an electronic format that makes the inevitable changes in the plan much easier. A third option may be found at www.Training Peaks.com, where a "VirtualCoach" will automatically create an ATP for you, using the same

instructions that follow. You may print it or use it online at this site, which offers many other services to self-coached athletes. Training Peaks charges a small monthly membership fee.

Fill in the blanks on the ATP, following these directions.

[Step 4: Put Dates on ATP]

Each of the rows on the ATP represents a week in the year. On the left side of the page, the column header "Wk# Mon" refers to the week number and the date of the Monday that week. The week numbers are already included; you just need to add the date for the Monday of each week of the season. For example, if you are starting your seasonal training for the year 2007 at the start of the new year, the date of the first Monday in January 2007 would be written in row 1, column 1 as "Jan 1." The second row would then be labeled "Jan 8" and the third "Jan 15." Repeat this pattern using a calendar to write in the consecutive Mondays for the entire season. Your training season may start at any point on the calendar, depending on when you are fully recovered from the previous season and when your races are scheduled for the coming season. It is best to allow at least 15 weeks to thoroughly prepare for your first A-priority race of the season. You may take as many as 32 weeks.

[Step 5: List Races]

Next, on your ATP, write in all of the events you intend to do in the coming season in the column labeled "Races." Place them on the ATP in the appropriate weeks, based on their dates. For example, let's say that you have an event scheduled for Saturday, January 13, 2007. It would be

PRIORITY	NUMBER IN A SEASON	DESCRIPTION	SPECIAL PREPARATION
A	1–3	Most important races. Your success is chiefly defined by their outcomes.	Taper for 2–3 weeks prior and follow Peak procedure.
B	4–8	Of secondary importance. You want to do well at these events, however.	Reduce training for 3–5 days before.
C	Unlimited—but be cautious!	Least important. Use as tune-ups, hard workouts, fun events, or growth as an athlete.	No special prep—treat these as workouts.

Table 9.1. Race Priorities

listed in the row marked "Jan 8" since that row includes all the dates from January 8 through January 14. If you have two events that same weekend, list them both in that row.

If unsure that you will do a particular race, list it anyway. It can be removed later. It is possible that you are completing this ATP several months in advance of the race season and the dates of events may not be published yet. In this case use the approximate date, based on when the event has been held in previous years.

[Step 6: Prioritize Races]

Once you have listed all your planned events, designate each as "A-priority," "B-priority," or "C-priority" by writing in A, B, or C in the "Pri" column next to the race name using the guidelines shown in Table 9.1. Most athletes designate nearly every event as A-priority. They want to be in top shape at all times. It just isn't possible. In fact, trying to peak for every event will only lead to reduced fitness and gradually worsening performances. Peaking for an A-priority race requires decreasing the training load and including more rest starting two to three weeks before the competition. If this is done too fre-

quently, your fitness will erode over the course of the season. Do not schedule more than two or three A-priorities in one season. Treat them as extraordinary occasions and prepare using the peaking procedure explained later in this chapter.

You must be cautious with the number of C-priority events. There is a psychological "cost" every time you toe a start line. Over-racing can easily result in burnout. C races are typically done for one of four reasons—as a tune-up before an A race, as a hard workout, as a social activity with friends, or as a learning experience. For novices, C races are a great way to learn more about the sport, so doing several the first year will speed up their growth as an athlete. Experienced athletes already know what the sport is like, so should have a very good reason for doing a C-priority event.

In the "Pri" column on your ATP write in the A-, B-, or C-priority for each event in the "Races" column.

[Step 7: Set Goals]

This is perhaps the most important part of completing your ATP, as it has a direct relation-

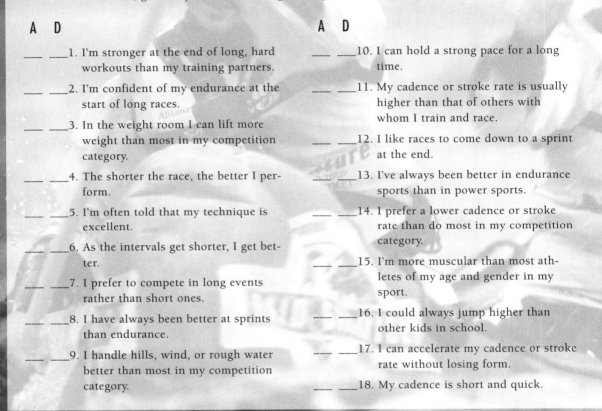

WHAT ARE YOUR WEAKNESSES?

Read each statement below and decide if you agree or disagree as it applies to you. Check the appropriate answer. If unsure, go with your initial feeling. A = Agree and D = Disagree.

A   D

___ ___ 1. I'm stronger at the end of long, hard workouts than my training partners.

___ ___ 2. I'm confident of my endurance at the start of long races.

___ ___ 3. In the weight room I can lift more weight than most in my competition category.

___ ___ 4. The shorter the race, the better I perform.

___ ___ 5. I'm often told that my technique is excellent.

___ ___ 6. As the intervals get shorter, I get better.

___ ___ 7. I prefer to compete in long events rather than short ones.

___ ___ 8. I have always been better at sprints than endurance.

___ ___ 9. I handle hills, wind, or rough water better than most in my competition category.

A   D

___ ___ 10. I can hold a strong pace for a long time.

___ ___ 11. My cadence or stroke rate is usually higher than that of others with whom I train and race.

___ ___ 12. I like races to come down to a sprint at the end.

___ ___ 13. I've always been better in endurance sports than in power sports.

___ ___ 14. I prefer a lower cadence or stroke rate than do most in my competition category.

___ ___ 15. I'm more muscular than most athletes of my age and gender in my sport.

___ ___ 16. I could always jump higher than other kids in school.

___ ___ 17. I can accelerate my cadence or stroke rate without losing form.

___ ___ 18. My cadence is short and quick.

ship to your satisfaction with the season when it is over. Give this a lot of thought.

The ATP provides spaces for three seasonal goals at the top of the page. I've found that three is about right for nearly every athlete. When there are too many goals, something gets neglected. You may have fewer, but no more than three.

You've probably heard this before, but it's worth repeating. Your goals should be well-defined by including two basic elements—what exactly you want to achieve and when you want

to achieve it. Goals should also be measurable. It isn't enough to set a goal of "Race faster." Goals should be more along the lines of this: "Complete the XYZ Race on May 7 in less than 40 minutes." The more tightly you define your goals, the easier you will find it is to work toward their successful accomplishment.

Goals should be event outcomes that are determined mostly by you rather than others. A goal to "Win the XYZ Race" has a lot to do with who is there that day and how fit they are. It is better to set a performance goal, such as a

A   D

___ ___ 19. I really like long, slow, easy workouts.

___ ___ 20. I was always pretty good at sports such as basketball, football, baseball, softball, or tennis.

___ ___ 21. I prefer a low cadence or stroke rate.

___ ___ 22. In school I could almost always beat the other kids in sprints.

___ ___ 23. To speed up, I accelerate my cadence or stroke rate.

___ ___ 24. I have some trouble in races if the pace accelerates frequently.

___ ___ 25. The longer the workout or race, the better I do.

___ ___ 26. I have great "lasting" ability in a race with a strong, steady pace but not great all-out speed.

___ ___ 27. I enjoy lifting weights.

___ ___ 28. I prefer workouts that are short, but fast.

___ ___ 29. My arm or leg turnover is quite high compared with that of most others in my sport.

___ ___ 30. I have always been able to throw, kick, or hit a ball farther than most others.

SCORING: For each of the following sets of statements, count and record the number of "Agree" answers you checked.

Statement numbers

2, 7, 13, 19, 25: Number of "Agrees" ____
Endurance score ____

3, 9, 15, 21, 27: Number of "Agrees" ____
Force score ____

5, 11, 17, 23, 29: Number of "Agrees" ____
Speed Skill score ____

1, 10, 14, 24, 26: Number of "Agrees" ____
Muscular Endurance score ____

4, 6, 18, 20, 28: Number of "Agrees" ____
Anaerobic Endurance score ____

8, 12, 16, 22, 30: Number of "Agrees" ____
Power score ____

time or strategy that you believe will win the race. The exception is when you know exactly who the competition is and what they are capable of doing in a race.

I once coached an athlete to race in the Olympic Trials for triathlon. He had to finish in at least third place to make the Olympic team, but the course was brand new and quite hilly and the weather hot and humid so we didn't know what time might accomplish that. However, we knew everyone who would be in the race and what to expect of them. So our

goal was to "Finish third or better at the Dallas Trials on May 28." He finished strongly in a come-from-behind third.

Make your goals event-outcome-oriented— how you want to do in the A-priority races. Almost everyone wants to set a goal of "Have fun!" That's commendable but assumed. If you're not a professional athlete who is trying to make money from the sport, fun is the only reason you're doing it. Fun is simply defined by people in different ways. For some it means being competitive; for others it has to do with socializing.

By all means, have fun, but also set race-performance goals that will stretch you as an athlete.

[Step 8: Determine Limiters]

By now your goal or goals should be listed at the top of the ATP. Can you achieve them? There should be at least a seed of doubt, otherwise the goal is too easy. If there is no question at all about your potential for success, then the goals aren't going to challenge you and training will have little purpose. When most effective, goals lie just beyond your current grasp. You should feel the need to train tenaciously and wisely to achieve them.

Here's something for you to ponder: Why can't you achieve your goals now? If you knew you could achieve them now, they would be accomplishments rather than goals, wouldn't they? Since

A-PRIORITY EVENT SUCCESS DETERMINERS

List your A-priority event or events.

Event 1: _____

Event 2: _____

Event 3: _____

Answer "yes" or "no" to each of the following questions for each event listed above.

ENDURANCE: To achieve my race goal, I must be able to finish what seems to me to be a very long distance.

Event #1   Yes_____ No_____

Event #2   Yes_____ No_____

Event #3   Yes_____ No_____

FORCE: To achieve my race goal, I must be able to go up hills, deal with strong headwinds, handle very rough water, or overcome some other form of resistance very strongly.

Event #1   Yes_____ No_____

Event #2   Yes_____ No_____

Event #3   Yes_____ No_____

SPEED SKILL: To achieve my race goal, I must be able to perform with a smooth and efficient technique—I can't afford to be even a little bit sloppy with my form.

Event #1   Yes_____ No_____

Event #2   Yes_____ No_____

Event #3   Yes_____ No_____

MUSCULAR ENDURANCE: To achieve my race goal, I must be able to maintain a moderately high, steady effort at the extreme edge of my capability for a long time.

Event #1   Yes_____ No_____

Event #2   Yes_____ No_____

Event #3   Yes_____ No_____

ANAEROBIC ENDURANCE: To achieve my race goal, I must be able to change pace frequently throughout the race, often greatly exceeding my lactate threshold heart rate.

Event #1   Yes_____ No_____

Event #2   Yes_____ No_____

Event #3   Yes_____ No_____

there is a bit of uncertainty about your performance capacity relative to your goals, obviously something is lacking that stands between you and immediate success. The purpose of your training is to "fix" this performance "limiter."

A limiter is a *race-specific* weakness. It's not merely a general weakness. For example, you may have a weakness when it comes to racing on hilly courses. But if your A-priority races are all flat, then this weakness is *not* a limiter. If we know what your limiters really are and train in such a way as to make them much stronger, then you will be able to achieve your goals. It's that simple.

The key question is: What are your limiters? Answering this question is the single most important thing you can do right now to move toward achieving your goals. Most athletes

POWER: To achieve my race goal, I must be able to sprint at maximum effort several times during the event or at the finish.

Event #1   Yes_____ No_____

Event #2   Yes_____ No_____

Event #3   Yes_____ No_____

SUMMARY: Determine the Training Triad demands for each of your A-priority events by checking off the abilities you indicated with "yes" above.

Event #1

_____ "Yes" for Endurance

_____ "Yes" for Force

_____ "Yes" for Speed Skill

_____ "Yes" for Muscular Endurance

_____ "Yes" for Anaerobic Endurance

_____ "Yes" for Power

Event #2

_____ "Yes" for Endurance

_____ "Yes" for Force

_____ "Yes" for Speed Skill

_____ "Yes" for Muscular Endurance

_____ "Yes" for Anaerobic Endurance

_____ "Yes" for Power

Event #3

_____ "Yes" for Endurance

_____ "Yes" for Force

_____ "Yes" for Speed Skill

_____ "Yes" for Muscular Endurance

_____ "Yes" for Anaerobic Endurance

_____ "Yes" for Power

never ask this question. They train absentmindedly, doing whatever is most enjoyable at the time. If they are good in the hills, they do lots of hill work. If endurance is their strength, they do mostly long workouts. Those who are blessed with great speed do short, fast workouts. It never dawns on these athletes that until they improve whatever it is that is holding them back they will never make a performance breakthrough. Continuing to focus on their strengths while giving lip service to their limiters means there will be little change in performance.

So, what *are* your limiters? The possibilities are endless, including everything that affects your athletic development in such broad categories as training, lifestyle, nutrition, time available for exercise, athletic equipment, training environment, support, susceptibility to illness and injury, poor tactics and strategy, lack of race experience, poor body composition, insufficient sleep, and psychological stress. While you need to examine yourself in terms of each of these categories, we will concern ourselves here primarily with training, and, even more specifically, the Training Triad described in Chapter 6.

Let's see if we can figure out what your strengths and weaknesses are in terms of the six abilities that make up the Training Triad. The "What Are Your Weaknesses?" sidebar on pages 118–19 will start you down the path to determining your limiters.

Recall from Chapter 6 that the Training Triad's abilities—endurance, force, speed skill, muscular endurance, anaerobic endurance, and power—are what determine how well you do physically in training and competition. The "What Are Your Weaknesses?" sidebar gives you a gauge of how you stack up in each of these six

abilities. The higher your score for a given ability, the more likely it is that the ability is one of your strengths and is something you should rely on when setting race strategy.

What we are most concerned with here, however, are your limiters. A score of 3 or less in any of the abilities indicates a weakness, but not necessarily a limiter. To determine whether a weakness is a limiter, you must compare it with what is demanded of your A-priority events in order to achieve your goals. Whenever an event demands a certain ability for success and you have a weakness in that ability, then you have a limiter. To determine what is required to achieve your performance goals for each A-priority competition you plan on doing, complete the questionnaire in the "A-Priority Event Success Determiners" sidebar.

The sidebar "A-Priority Event Success Determiners" on pages 120–21 tells you which abilities are required for success in your A-priority events. By comparing event success requirements with your weaknesses from the earlier sidebar, limiters are determined. This in turn indicates where your training focus needs to be. For example, if you determined in this chapter's first sidebar that a weakness you have is muscular endurance and the second sidebar indicates that at least one of your events requires good muscular endurance for success, then this ability is a limiter for you. You should now be able to identify your limiters using a third sidebar, titled "What Are Your Limiters?"

[Step 9: Establish Training Objectives]

Let's use an old analogy to understand what this is all about. A chain (your performance) is only as strong as its weakest link (your limiter). A chain will always break at its weakest link. Making all the other links stronger does no good—the chain continues to break at the weak link. Until the weak link is made stronger, the entire chain is weak. Make that one link stronger, however, and the whole chain gets stronger.

In like manner, the things you need to accomplish in training in order to strengthen your "weak links"—your limiters—are called "training objectives." Strengthen these links by achieving certain objectives in training, and your performance takes a great leap forward. Ignore them and you will always "break" at the same place in A-priority races.

There are five lines at the top of the ATP where the objectives of your training are to be listed. This can be a real head scratcher. Let's see if we can figure it out.

You now know from the sidebar on limiters what your limiters are. So the first question is: What do you do about them? The answer, of course, is to "fix" them. Even with concentrated training, it's unlikely that in one season they will become your greatest strengths (a score of "5" on the weaknesses sidebar), but you need to

WHAT ARE YOUR LIMITERS?

By comparing the results of the first two sidebars in this chapter, I know that my Training Triad ability limiters are (check each that applies to you):

_____ Endurance

_____ Force

_____ Speed Skill

_____ Muscular Endurance

_____ Anaerobic Endurance

_____ Power

In addition, I believe my other limiters are (check any that apply to you):

_____ My lifestyle is not conducive to good training.

_____ My nutrition is poor.

_____ My time available for exercise is inadequate.

_____ My athletic equipment is outdated or otherwise inadequate.

_____ My training environment (weather, terrain, access to training facilities) is inadequate.

_____ I receive little support from my family and friends for my training and racing.

_____ I catch colds easily.

_____ I get injured easily.

_____ I have a tendency to overtrain.

_____ My race tactics and strategy are poorly planned or implemented.

_____ I lack race experience.

_____ My body composition is holding me back.

_____ I get insufficient sleep.

_____ I experience a lot of psychological stress.

ABILITY	HOW TO TRAIN THE ABILITY
Endurance	Long, steady workouts done in Zone 2, especially its upper half.
Force	Weight lifting or other strength training. Resisted (hills, tethers, drag devices), sport-specific workouts done with short (<2 minutes) intervals in Zones 3 and 4 and long recoveries.
Speed Skill	Very short repeats done at high cadence or stroke rate with long recoveries. High frequency important. Too brief for heart rate to be an effective intensity gauge.
Muscular Endurance	Long (6–12 minutes) intervals with short recoveries; or long (20–60 minutes), steady efforts done in Zones 3, 4, and 5a.
Anaerobic Endurance	Short (2–4 minutes), fast intervals with about equal recovery durations done in Zone 5b.
Power	Very short (less than 20 seconds) sprint intervals with long recovery durations (several minutes) at Zone 5c effort (so short that heart rate may not be effective).

Table 9.2. How to Train the Abilities

start moving in that direction. How can you do that? Simple. You need to devote more training to your limiting abilities than you are doing now. And how do you train the abilities that are your limiters? This was explained in Chapter 6. Table 9.2 summarizes how to train each ability. For more details see Tables 6.1 and 6.2. Appendix 5 provides specific workouts for each ability.

The objectives to be listed on your ATP could be referred to as "sub-goals"—things you must accomplish in training to show that you are making progress toward correcting your limiters. Since you now know what your limiters are and the types of workouts you will do to make these abilities stronger, you need to know when you've made measurable progress. That's why you have training objectives.

You'll be tempted to skip this part of the ATP because it requires deep thought and painstaking analysis. Don't overlook this section. If you do, your training plan will never have the focus needed to really kickstart your athletic performance. This step gives a deeper meaning to all the work you have done so far as well as a focused direction to your training.

The following are some examples of training objectives, listed by ability. These may give you some ideas about what yours might be. Give this some thought and then list your training objectives at the top of your ATP. There is room for five. You'll need at least one objective for each limiter. Be sure to indicate when you anticipate achieving the objective. This date should be in advance of your A-priority race for which that improved ability is needed for success.

Endurance Objective examples

- Within a 6-week period complete 6, 4-hour workouts in Zone 2 with the last on July 8.

- Maintain coupling of high AeT heart rate and pace for 2 hours by the end of the Base period.

Force Objective examples

- Freebar squat 1.5 × body weight by January 7.

- Average over 400 watts for 1-minute climb on 8% grade by January 14.

Speed Skill Objective examples

- Complete a 5k race with an average cadence of 88 by August 12.

- Complete a 1000-meter time trial with an average cadence of 45 to 55 by February 4.

Muscular Endurance Objective examples

- Take 30 seconds off my self-test TTT time at heart rate range 141 to 143 by September 2.

- Improve pace by 20 seconds for 1 mile at Zone 5a by August 12.

Anaerobic Endurance Objective examples

- Complete 15 minutes of Zone 5b intervals at an average pace of under 6 minutes by August 19.

- Complete a 1.5-mile time trial faster than 10 minutes by June 17.

Power Objective examples

- Sprint up Bell Road hill in under 10 seconds from a standing start by June 24.

- Increase maximum instantaneous power to more than 1000 watts by May 6.

[Step 10: Assign Mesocycles]

You'll be glad to know that the hard part, the part that makes your brain hurt, is now done. What remains is far less thought-provoking but no less important. The next task in completing your ATP is to periodize your season. That means assigning mesocycle periods to each week of the year.

In Chapter 8 you learned about the six mesocycles—Prep, Base, Build, Peak, Race, and Transition. Table 8.1 provided a summary of these periods, showing how long each mesocycle lasts, what the purpose is, and what Training Triad abilities are emphasized in each. You may want to glance at that table once again to refresh your memory before completing this portion of your ATP.

In the column marked "Period" you will write in the name of the mesocycle assigned to each week. You'll do this by working backward from each of your A-priority races. As Table 8.1 shows, there is a range of weeks for each mesocycle. For example, the Base period is 6 to 12 weeks long. How do you decide the duration of your mesocycle, given such wide ranges? There are two parts to the answer.

The first part is that when preparing for your first A race of the season you should always schedule at the high end of each range, especially when it comes to the Base period. You are more likely to do 12 rather than 6 weeks of Base early in the season. For subsequent A races in the season, the lower end of each range is more commonly used since your fitness is fairly well established from months of prior training. Later in the season, when preparing for a second or third A race, the Base period may even be omitted. More on that later.

The second part of the answer to how many weeks should be included for each mesocycle is a bit more complex and more or less involves your age. It actually has to do with your capacity for recovery, but this is largely determined by how many years you've been on the planet. Young athletes generally recover more quickly than older athletes and therefore may schedule longer mesocycles. That means young athletes will have more days or weeks of challenging training before taking a rest and recovery (R&R) break. Older athletes need these breaks more frequently, since they are more easily overtrained.

Some of the mesocycles are made up of sub-periods. For example, the entire Base period is made up of Base 1, Base 2, and Base 3, while the Build mesocycle has sub-periods Build 1 and Build 2. The Base and Build sub-periods each end with several days of R&R. The athlete trains hard for several days and then rests for a few days. While the young athlete trains hard for about three weeks before taking a few days of R&R, the older athlete only goes hard for about two weeks before taking a break.

So, I know what you're thinking: "What does 'older' mean?" While it may be explained by age, it is better defined by your capacity for recovery. I've known 35-year-olds who recovered slowly, and I've also known athletes who were 55 yet recovered quickly. A quick gauge of which category you fall into may be determined by how you spring back after an anaerobic endurance workout. If after doing 15 minutes or more of intervals in Zone 5b you find it typically takes you more than 2 days to be ready to go hard again, then you are an older athlete regardless of your age. If unsure about this simple test, just use your age until you get a better gauge. If

PERIOD	YOUNG ATHLETE	OLDER ATHLETE
Prep	2–6 weeks	2–6 weeks
Base 1	4 weeks	3 weeks
Base 2	4 weeks	3 weeks
Base 3	4 weeks	3 weeks (repeat)
Build 1	4 weeks	3 weeks
Build 2	4 weeks	3 weeks (repeat)
Peak	1–2 weeks	1–2 weeks
Race	1–2 weeks	1–2 weeks
Transition	1–4 weeks	1–4 weeks

Table 9.3. Mesocycle Sub-period Durations by Age Category

you are under 45, assume you are young, and if beyond that age let's classify you as older for the purposes of completing your ATP for now.

Once we know your age category, we can decide how long your sub-periods of each mesocycle are. Table 9.3 summarizes the period durations by age.

Notice that the older athlete repeats Base 3 and Build 2, thus doing 12 weeks of Base training (4 sub-periods of 3 weeks each) and 9 weeks of Build (3 sub-periods of 3 weeks each). The young athlete also does 12 weeks of Base but only 8 of Build—1 week less. The older athlete needs that extra week of hard training because this mesocycle tends to be the most challenging, so spreading it out a bit over a longer time frame is beneficial for the athlete who doesn't recover quickly.

With all this in mind, it's time to complete the "Period" column on your ATP. You'll fill in this column by working backward. Start with the first A-priority race of the season. At the intersection of the Period column and appropriate A-race row, write in "Race." Then count up two rows and write in "Peak" for both of these weeks. The next two mesocycles vary, based on your age category. (Take another look at the sample Annual Training Plan on pages 114–15 if unsure about the procedure so far.)

If you have classified yourself as a young athlete, count up four weeks and write in "Build 2" for each of these weeks. Again, count up four weeks and write in "Build 1." Do the same for Base 3, Base 2, and Base 1. If you are an older athlete, assign three weeks to each of these periods.

Then the top two to six weeks are labeled "Prep" regardless of your athletic age. How many of these you schedule depends on when your previous season ended and how ready you are to start focused training again. If unsure that you are ready, it's best to take some more time off.

Finally, the week after your first A race write in "Tran"—short for Transition. If this first Transition mesocycle comes early in your season, then I'd strongly suggest that you take a few days off from training. This may only be 3 to 7 days. The idea is to give not only your body but also your mind a break. Feel free to just goof off for a few days. But if you can't stand the thought of not exercising, just do one short workout in Zone 1 daily. Keep in mind, though, that the purpose here is to rest and rejuvenate by not having a routine or workouts that *must* be done.

The first macrocycle on the season is now complete. It was the easy one. Basically, we just followed a formula to plan it. For the subsequent macrocycles, you have a few decisions to make and some mesocycles that are left out.

For example, when scheduling beyond the first A race, you will not repeat the Prep period and probably not Base 1 or Base 2 either. However, you may want to return to Base 3 after the first Transition period if your basic abilities (endurance, force, or speed skill) have declined in the last few weeks. This is not unusual following a long Peak and race period. You may even want to do Base 3 twice, if you have enough weeks. If your basic abilities, especially endurance, are lacking, then that will greatly detract from training and racing the rest of the season. But if your basic abilities are still strong, you may want to start back into training with a Build 1 or Build 2 period. But don't shortchange the basic abilities in order to do more high heart rate training.

Using the sample Annual Training Plan on pages 114–15 as a model, finish filling in the "Period" column on your ATP through the end of the season. Later on, should you decide that the plan you have isn't right, you can always make changes. I've coached very few athletes who made it all the way through a season with no ATP adjustments.

[Step 11: Set Weekly Training Hours]

As you can see, we're working our way down to more and more detailed aspects of your training. You've now got most of the ATP complete and we have a general idea of what you will do in training. What remains are the specifics, such as setting the number of hours you will work out weekly—your volume. Once volume is determined, you're ready to take care of the final details—the actual workouts.

Weekly volume is the product of duration and frequency—how long and how often you work out. For example, if you work out for two hours each day and 7 days a week, your volume is 14 hours. Setting volume is done in one of two ways. You either determine how many weekly hours you have available for training or you decide the seasonal volume ("Annual Hours" at the top of the ATP) necessary to achieve your goals.

The first is the easier to figure out. You simply subtract all the weekly commitments and demands on your time from 168, the number of hours in a week. To compute your available training hours for each week, see the sidebar titled "How Many Training Hours Do You Have?" If you're a busy person, as most athletes are, this little exercise will tell you the average number of weekly hours you have available for training. Multiply the result by 50 and you know approximately how many annual hours you can train. That number is placed at the top of the ATP where it says "Annual Hours."

If your available training hours are fewer than you believe you could handle each week, then setting your weekly hours for the season is pretty easy. Simply schedule the time you have available for each week, with the exception of R&R and "Race" weeks every third or fourth week (depending on your training-age category as explained in Step 10). Write your training hours for each non-R&R and "Race" week of the season in the "Hours" column on your ATP (refer to the sample Annual Training Plan on pages 114–15 for guidance). For the R&R weeks, figure you will train from 60 to 80 percent of whatever your available hours are. Where you fit in this range depends on how close you are to your physical volume limit in the other weeks. If quite close—in other words, the other weeks are likely to leave you quite tired even though you could have done a bit more if there were more hours available—then make the R&R weeks 60 percent of a "normal" week. If you know you could handle a lot more

HOW MANY TRAINING HOURS DO YOU HAVE?

Everyone, no matter how busy, has 168 hours available each week of the year. We can choose to use the hours in any way we want. For athletes, some hours need to be devoted to working out. How are *your* 168 hours used each week? Below, estimate how many hours are spent in each nonexercise category each week.

Sleep	_____
Work	_____
Eat	_____

Family time	_____
Personal hygiene	_____
Housework	_____
Home maintenance	_____
Goofing off (TV, etc.)	_____
Other (nonexercise)	_____
Total Hours Spent	_____
Training Hours (168 minus Total Hours Spent)	_____

PERIOD	WEEK	200	250	300	350	400	450	500	550	600	650	700	750	800	850	900	950	1000
Prep	All	3.5	4.0	5.0	6.0	7.0	7.5	8.5	9.0	10.0	11.0	12.0	12.5	13.5	14.5	15.0	16.0	17.0
Base 1	1	4.0	5.0	6.0	7.0	8.0	9.0	10.0	11.0	12.0	12.5	14.0	14.5	15.5	16.5	17.5	18.5	19.5
	2	5.0	6.0	7.0	8.5	9.5	10.5	12.0	13.0	14.5	15.5	16.5	18.0	19.0	20.0	21.5	22.5	24.0
	3	5.5	6.5	8.0	9.5	10.5	12.0	13.5	14.5	16.0	17.5	18.5	20.0	21.5	22.5	24.0	25.5	26.5
	4	3.0	3.5	4.0	5.0	5.5	6.5	7.0	8.0	8.5	9.0	10.0	10.5	11.5	12.0	12.5	13.5	14.0
Base 2	1	4.0	5.5	6.5	7.5	8.5	9.5	10.5	12.5	12.5	13.0	14.5	16.0	17.0	18.0	19.0	20.0	21.0
	2	5.0	6.5	7.5	9.0	10.0	11.5	12.5	14.0	15.0	16.5	17.5	19.0	20.0	21.5	22.5	24.0	25.0
	3	5.5	7.0	8.5	10.0	11.0	12.5	14.0	15.5	17.0	18.0	19.5	21.0	22.5	24.0	25.0	26.5	28.0
	4	4.0	5.5	6.5	7.5	8.5	9.5	10.5	12.5	12.5	13.0	14.5	16.0	17.0	18.0	19.0	20.0	21.0
Base 3	1	4.5	5.5	7.0	8.0	9.0	10.0	11.0	12.5	13.5	14.5	15.5	17.0	18.0	19.0	20.0	21.0	22.5
	2	5.0	6.5	8.0	9.5	10.5	12.0	13.5	14.5	16.0	17.0	18.5	20.0	21.5	23.0	24.0	25.0	26.5
	3	6.0	7.5	9.0	10.5	11.5	13.0	15.0	16.5	18.0	19.0	20.5	22.0	23.5	25.0	26.5	28.0	29.5
	4	4.0	5.5	6.5	7.5	8.5	9.5	10.5	12.5	12.5	13.0	14.5	16.0	17.0	18.0	19.0	20.0	21.0
Build 1	1	5.0	6.5	8.0	9.0	10.0	11.5	12.5	14.0	15.5	16.0	17.5	19.0	20.5	21.5	22.5	24.0	25.0
	2	5.0	6.5	8.0	9.0	10.0	11.5	12.5	14.0	15.5	16.0	17.5	19.0	20.5	21.5	22.5	24.0	25.0
	3	5.0	6.5	8.0	9.0	10.0	11.5	12.5	14.0	15.5	16.0	17.5	19.0	20.5	21.5	22.5	24.0	25.0
	4	4.0	5.5	6.5	7.5	8.5	9.5	10.5	12.5	12.5	13.0	14.5	16.0	17.0	18.0	19.0	20.0	21.0
Build 2	1	5.0	6.0	7.0	8.5	9.5	10.5	12.0	13.0	14.5	15.5	16.5	18.0	19.0	20.5	21.5	22.5	24.0
	2	5.0	6.0	7.0	8.5	9.5	10.5	12.0	13.0	14.5	15.5	16.5	18.0	19.0	20.5	21.5	22.5	24.0
	3	5.0	6.0	7.0	8.5	9.5	10.5	12.0	13.0	14.5	15.5	16.5	18.0	19.0	20.5	21.5	22.5	24.0
	4	4.0	5.5	6.5	7.5	8.5	9.5	10.5	12.5	12.5	13.0	14.5	16.0	17.0	18.0	19.0	20.0	21.0
Peak	1	4.0	5.5	6.5	7.5	8.5	9.5	10.5	11.5	13.0	13.5	14.5	16.0	17.0	18.0	19.0	20.0	21.0
	2	3.5	4.0	5.0	6.0	6.5	7.5	8.5	9.5	10.0	11.0	11.5	12.5	13.5	14.5	15.0	16.0	17.0
Race	All	4.0	5.5	6.5	7.5	8.5	9.5	10.5	12.5	12.5	13.0	14.5	16.0	17.0	18.0	19.0	20.0	21.0

Table 9.5. Weekly Training Hours

A-PRIORITY RACE DURATION	ANNUAL VOLUME FOR GOAL OF "FINISH THE RACE"	ANNUAL VOLUME FOR GOAL OF "HIGH PERFORMANCE"
Up to 3 hours	200–400	500–1,000
3 to 8 hours	300–500	600–1,000
More than 8 hours	450–600	700–1,000

Table 9.4. Suggested Annual Volume Based on Race Duration and Race Goal

hours than are available to you, then multiply by 80 percent to set R&R weekly hours. Obviously, there is a lot of guessing going on here, so you could use some other multiplier between 60 and 70 percent if that seems appropriate.

How much training time do you schedule if the demands on your time are not restrictive? To answer this, you need to first understand annual training hours, or how much time you devote to training in an entire year. Once we know that number, you can schedule the time for each mesocycle based on what has been shown to work for other athletes.

Your annual hours includes everything you do in all workouts intended to improve your Training Triad abilities from Chapter 6. Besides your sport-specific workouts, this includes strength training and all cross training activities. Use Table 9.4 to help you decide what your annual volume should be. This table is based on the duration of your longest A-priority event and the level of your season's goals. For the sake of simplicity, the goals are divided into "finish the race" and "high performance." The first is easy to understand. The second is defined only by your aspirations relative to your known level of performance. If achieving your goals is going to push you to your physical limits, then they are high performance.

There is a lot of wiggle room in the suggested annual volume ranges in Table 9.4. It's best, though, not to increase your hours from one year to the next by more than 15 percent. So select a number from the appropriate range that is only slightly more than what you have done in past seasons.

Record your Annual Volume at the top of the ATP. To set weekly hours, find your annual volume in the top row of Table 9.5. Using this table you may now complete the "Hours" column on your ATP. For example, if annual volume is 400 hours, then the Prep period is 7.0 hours; Base 1, week 1 is 8.0 hours; and Base 1, week 2 is 9.5 hours.

[Step 12: Schedule Heart Rate-Based Workouts]

Appendix 4 suggests weekly microcycle patterns for various types of endurance sports, according to your level of experience and the mesocycle. Appendix 5 provides a sampling of heart rate–based workouts by Training Triad abilities. In this step you will combine these two to fit your exact needs by matching training with your limiters, strengths, weekly routine, and time available.

Turn to Appendix 4 and select the weekly microcycle training pattern for each mesocycle

WEEKLY HOURS	SUGGESTED DAILY HOURS					
3.0	1.0	0.75	0.75	0.5	0	0	0
3.5	1.5	0.75	0.75	0.5	0	0	0
4.0	1.5	1.0	1.0	0.5	0	0	0
4.5	1.5	1.0	0.75	0.75	0.5	0	0
5.0	1.5	1.0	1.0	1.0	0.5	0	0
5.5	1.5	1.25	1.0	1.0	0.75	0	0
6.0	1.5	1.25	1.0	1.0	0.75	0.5	0
6.5	1.5	1.25	1.0	1.0	1.0	0.75	0
7.0	1.5	1.5	1.25	1.0	1.0	0.75	0
7.5	2.0	1.5	1.25	1.0	1.0	0.75	0
8.0	2.0	1.5	1.25	1.25	1.0	1.0	0
8.5	2.0	1.5	1.25	1.25	1.0	1.0	0.5
9.0	2.0	1.5	1.5	1.25	1.0	1.0	0.75
9.5	2.5	1.5	1.5	1.25	1.0	1.0	0.75
10.0	2.5	2.0	1.5	1.25	1.0	1.0	0.75
10.5	2.5	2.0	1.5	1.5	1.0	1.0	1.0
11.0	2.5	2.0	1.5	1.5	1.5	1.0	1.0
11.5	3.0	2.0	1.5	1.5	1.5	1.0	1.0
12.0	3.0	2.0	2.0	1.5	1.5	1.0	1.0
12.5	3.5	2.0	2.0	1.5	1.5	1.0	1.0
13.0	3.5	2.5	2.0	1.5	1.5	1.0	1.0
13.5	3.5	2.5	2.0	2.0	1.5	1.0	1.0
14.0	4.0	2.5	2.0	2.0	1.5	1.0	1.0
14.5	4.0	2.5	2.0	2.0	1.5	1.5	1.0
15.0	4.0	2.5	2.5	2.0	1.5	1.5	1.0
15.5	4.0	2.5	2.5	2.0	2.0	1.5	1.0
16.0	4.0	3.0	2.5	2.0	2.0	1.5	1.0
16.5	4.0	3.0	2.5	2.5	2.0	1.5	1.0
17.0	4.0	3.0	2.5	2.5	2.0	2.0	1.0
17.5	4.5	3.0	3.0	2.5	2.0	2.0	1.0
18.0	4.5	3.0	3.0	2.5	2.5	2.0	1.0
18.5	4.5	3.0	3.0	2.5	2.5	2.0	1.0
19.0	4.5	3.5	3.0	2.5	2.5	2.0	1.0
19.5	4.5	3.5	3.0	3.0	2.5	2.0	1.0
20.0	4.5	3.5	3.0	3.0	2.5	2.5	1.0
20.5	5.0	3.5	3.0	3.0	2.5	2.5	1.0
21.0	5.0	3.5	3.5	3.0	2.5	2.5	1.0
21.5	5.0	3.5	3.5	3.0	3.0	2.5	1.0
22.0	5.0	4.0	3.5	3.0	3.0	2.5	1.0
22.5	5.0	4.0	3.5	3.5	3.0	2.5	1.0
23.0	5.0	4.0	3.5	3.5	3.0	2.5	1.5
23.5	5.5	4.0	3.5	3.5	3.0	2.5	1.5
24.0	5.5	4.0	4.0	3.5	3.0	2.5	1.5
24.5	5.5	4.0	4.0	3.5	3.5	2.5	1.5
25.0	5.5	4.5	4.0	3.5	3.5	2.5	1.5
25.5	5.5	4.5	4.0	4.0	3.5	2.5	1.5
26.0	6.0	4.5	4.0	4.0	3.5	2.5	1.5
26.5	6.0	4.5	4.0	4.0	3.5	3.0	1.5
27.0	6.0	4.5	4.5	4.0	3.5	3.0	1.5
27.5	6.0	4.5	4.5	4.0	4.0	3.0	1.5
28.0	6.0	5.0	4.5	4.0	4.0	3.0	1.5
28.5	6.0	5.0	4.5	4.5	4.0	3.0	1.5
29.0	6.0	5.0	4.5	4.5	4.0	3.5	1.5
29.5	6.0	5.0	4.5	4.5	4.0	3.5	2.0
30.0	6.0	5.0	5.0	4.5	4.0	3.5	2.0
30.5	6.0	5.0	5.0	4.5	4.5	3.5	2.0
31.0	6.0	5.5	5.0	4.5	4.5	3.5	2.0

Table 9.6. Daily Training Hours

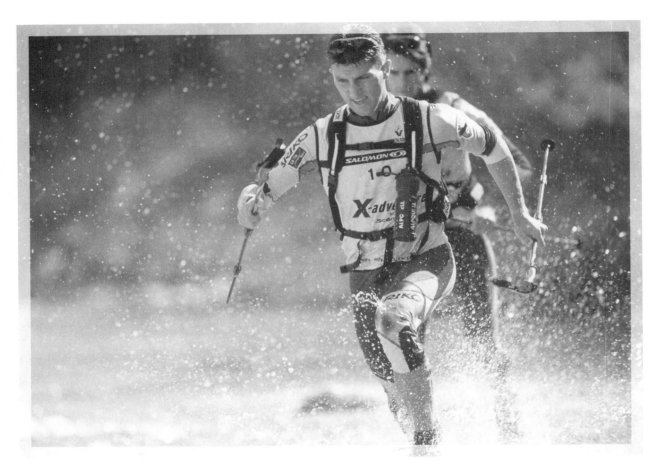

of the season that best matches your experience level and type of sport (steady state or variably paced). Then, for each microcycle pattern, select the exact workouts you will do each day from Appendix 5. Note that the workouts in Appendix 5 are coded. Simply write the codes for the workouts you've selected in the daily spaces for the rows marked as "Workout Codes."

All that now remains is to set a training time for each workout. This is done using Table 9.6. The "Hours" column on your ATP indicates how much training time is planned for each week. Take the time for a given week and find that same number in the "Weekly Hours" column of Table 9.6. By reading across the seven columns to the right of that number, you'll see how to distribute the time for each day of the week. For example, let's say your hours for a given week on your ATP are 8.0. The seven times to the right of that are 2.0, 1.5, 1.25, 1.25, 1.0, 1.0, and 0. This tells you how many hours to work out each day when you have 8 hours planned for a week. You may put those times on whichever days work best for you. If you are using Appendix 4, the figures suggest daily duration levels. The daily hours stay the same whether you are doing one workout a day or multiple workouts. For example, if you are doing two-a-days and have 2.0 hours planned for that day, you could do 2, 1-hour workouts.

Once all this is done, your training is a breeze—well, except for the actual work. All you need to do each week is glance ahead to the coming week to see what's planned.

I mentioned earlier in this chapter that you should expect your ATP to change in reaction to illness, race date changes, and other unforeseen occurrences. That's why the ATP should be done either in pencil or in an electronic format. When these inevitable changes happen, simply return to this chapter and make the needed adjustments. Such changes usually mean losing some training time and fitness. Whatever you do, don't try to make up for such losses by doubling up on the workouts. This will only lead to greater problems down the road.

THE HEART OF THE MATTER

This chapter took you through the 12-step planning process that I use in coaching athletes. By building a plan using this process, you have designed your entire season based precisely on your unique needs. All that remains is to do the workouts. Having and following a detailed plan increases your confidence, which in turn improves performance. With this plan you're well on your way to achieving your goals.

If you'd prefer not to go through all the detail suggested here, you can find generic, 12-week mesocycles at www.TargetHRT.com for running, cycling, triathlon, duathlon, and mountain biking, categorized by experience level. Click on "Training Plans." Or you can become a member at www.TrainingPeaks.com and have the "VirtualCoach" there fill out all the worksheets and make all these decisions for you, based on information you provide. There are small fees for both TargetHRT.com training plans and TrainingPeaks.com membership. Whichever you do, it is imperative that you follow the plan and use your heart rate to guide the intensity of all workouts.

APPENDICES

COMMON FIELD TESTS FOR LACTATE THRESHOLD HEART RATE

The following are self-tests you can do to determine lactate threshold (LT) heart rate for your sport. Once you know your LT heart rate, set up your heart rate training zones by finding your sport's heart rate table in Appendix 2. Find your LT heart rate in the bold numbers in the "5a" column. Reading the row both left and right of this number produces your heart rate zones.

[30-Minute Test]

This is a simple test—but not easy. All you have to do is complete a 30-minute time trial on a constant course, such as a flat road, slight uphill, or calm water. It may also be done indoors on an ergometer for your sport, such as a bike trainer, rower, or treadmill. Most athletes find this harder to do indoors than outdoors. If you decide to test indoors, be sure to have a fan or cool room to exercise in. Heat will adversely affect results. This test is best done alone, as having a partner may also affect the results.

Start by warming up adequately. You should have a sense of what that means for you, since it should be about the same as what you do before a race. Most athletes need at least 10 minutes of warm-up before this test. But you may want as much as 30 minutes.

Once warmed up and ready to go, immediately start the test. The key to this test is pacing. Almost everyone starts at too great an intensity and then fades in the last few minutes. It's not unusual to hear of athletes failing to finish the test the first time because they started out too

fast. Tell yourself you'll hold back just a little the first 10 minutes, and continually remind yourself of this once the test begins.

At exactly 10 minutes into the test, click the lap button on your heart rate monitor. Then when the test ends, click the stop button. You now will have three heart rate-data points captured on your heart rate monitor—average heart rate for the first 10 minutes, average for the last 20 minutes, and average for the entire 30 minutes. The one we are interested in is your average for the last 20 minutes. This provides a good estimate of your LT heart rate. Use it to determine your heart rate zones, as described in Chapter 3.

Other good information to record from this test is your average velocity or power for the entire 30 minutes. For while your LT heart rate might not change much in subsequent tests, with improving fitness both velocity and power *will* change for the better.

Using the 30-minute self-test, my LT heart rate is estimated as _____.

[Graded Exercise Test]

This test is similar to what you would do in a test in a clinic or lab, but, of course, does not include the use of expensive metabolic assessment equipment. Besides a heart rate monitor, you will need an ergometer that's appropriate for your sport. This could be a treadmill for running, a stationary bike or indoor bicycle trainer, or a rowing ergometer. (This test does not work well for swimming unless you use a flume.) The ergometer must accurately display some output measure such as speed, pace, or watts. Be sure that the ergometer is set for the "manual" mode. You will also need an assistant to hold the heart rate monitor receiver (wristwatch) and to record information.

The following is a description of how to conduct the test.

1. Warm up on the equipment for 10 to 15 minutes.

2. Set the machine to start the test at a very easy resistance—something that takes little effort to do. Your RPE should be on the low end in the first minute—about 2 on the 1- to-10 scale described in Chapter 3 (you might place the RPE page where it can be seen during the test).

3. Every minute, increase the machine's resistance by a small amount. Your effort level will rise steadily. This continues until you are forced to stop because of fatigue.

4. Each minute, your assistant records the current level of output (speed, pace, power). At the end of each minute, tell your assistant how great your exertion is, using the 1-to- 10 RPE scale.

5. Your assistant records your exertion rating and your heart rate at the end of the minute and assists you, if necessary, in changing the equipment to the next higher level of resistance.

6. The assistant also listens closely to your breathing to detect when it first becomes deep and forceful. This is the "VT," or ventilatory threshold, which correlates quite closely with lactate threshold. The more times your assistant helps you conduct this test, the better he or she will get at identifying the VT.

7. Continue the test by increasing the resistance every minute until you can no longer hold the output.

The following is an example of the data collected from such a test. The "Output" column is not specific to any particular sport or ergometer. Your numbers may well be different for each column, but this is generally the way it will look.

Output	Heart Rate	RPE
1.5	110	2
2.0	118	3
2.5	125	3
3.0	135	4
3.5	142	5
4.0	147	6
4.5	153	6
5.0	156	7 "VT"
5.5	159	7
6.0	163	8
6.5	165	9

Now that you have collected the data, it's time to locate your approximate lactate threshold (LT) heart rate. Use the following guidelines to do that.

1. If you really pushed yourself, your LT heart rate will be found in the last five data points. In the example above, the last five data points begin with an output of "4.5."

2. If an RPE of 7 is found in the last five data points, assume that where it first appears is your LT heart rate. If you did not push yourself to your limit on the test, assume

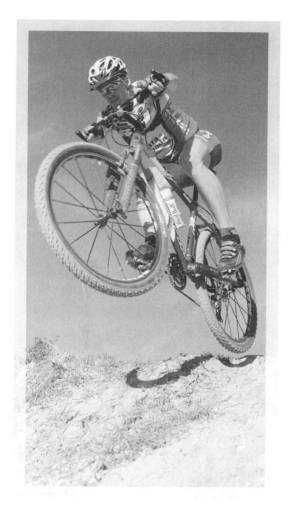

Applying these criteria to the example above, the LT heart rate is found to be 156 bpm. Realize that this is merely an estimate of your LT heart rate. You may get slightly different results with subsequent tests. But for now use this number to determine your heart rate zones, as described in Chapter 3.

Using the graded-exercise self-test, my LT heart rate is estimated as _____.

that where you assigned a 7 RPE is your LT heart rate.

3. If RPE 7 occurs before the last five data points and your assistant's subjective identification of VT is found in that range, assume that this is your LT heart rate.

4. If neither RPE 7 nor your assistant's VT notation is found in the last five data points, then assume that your LT heart rate is the fifth one before the end of the test.

CYCLING, ROWING, INLINE SKATING
HEART RATE ZONES

Find your LT heart rate **(bold)** in the "Zone 5a" column. Read across, left and right, for training zones.

ZONE 1: Active Recovery   ZONE 2: Aerobic Threshold   ZONE 3: Tempo   ZONE 4: Sub-Lactate Threshold
ZONE 5A: Lactate Threshold   ZONE 5B: Aerobic Capacity   ZONE 5C: Anaerobic Capacity

ZONE 1	ZONE 2	ZONE 3	ZONE 4	ZONE 5A	ZONE 5B	ZONE 5C
<109	109–122	123–128	129–136	**137–140**	141–145	146+
<110	110–123	124–129	130–137	**138–141**	142–146	147+
<110	110–124	125–130	131–138	**139–142**	143–147	148+
<111	111–125	126–130	131–139	**140–143**	144–147	148+
<112	112–125	126–131	132–140	**141–144**	145–148	149+
<113	113–126	127–132	133–141	**142–145**	146–149	150+
<113	113–127	128–133	134–142	**143–145**	146–150	151+
<114	114–128	129–134	135–143	**144–147**	148–151	152+
<115	115–129	130–135	136–144	**145–148**	149–152	153+
<116	116–130	131–136	137–145	**146–149**	150–154	155+
<117	117–131	132–137	138–146	**147–150**	151–155	156+
<118	118–132	133–138	139–147	**148–151**	152–156	157+
<119	119–133	134–139	140–148	**149–152**	153–157	158+
<120	120–134	135–140	141–149	**150–153**	154–158	159+
<121	121–134	135–141	142–150	**151–154**	155–159	160+
<122	122–135	136–142	143–151	**152–155**	156–160	161+
<123	123–136	137–142	143–152	**153–156**	157–161	162+
<124	124–137	138–143	144–153	**154–157**	158–162	163+
<125	125–138	139–144	145–154	**155–158**	159–163	164+
<126	126–138	139–145	146–155	**156–159**	160–164	165+
<127	127–140	141–146	147–156	**157–160**	161–165	166+
<128	128–141	142–147	148–157	**158–161**	162–167	168+
<129	129–142	143–148	149–158	**159–162**	163–168	169+
<130	130–143	144–148	149–159	**160–163**	164–169	170+
<130	130–143	144–150	151–160	**161–164**	165–170	171+
<131	131–144	145–151	152–161	**162–165**	166–171	172+

APPENDIX 2

ZONE 1	ZONE 2	ZONE 3	ZONE 4	ZONE 5A	ZONE 5B	ZONE 5C
<132	132–145	146–152	153–162	**163**–166	167–172	173+
<133	133–146	147–153	154–163	**164**–167	168–173	174+
<134	134–147	148–154	155–164	**165**–168	169–174	175+
<135	135–148	149–154	155–165	**166**–169	170–175	176+
<136	136–149	150–155	156–166	**167**–170	171–176	177+
<137	137–150	151–156	157–167	**168**–171	172–177	178+
<138	138–151	152–157	158–168	**169**–172	173–178	179+
<139	139–151	152–158	159–169	**170**–173	174–179	180+
<140	140–152	153–160	161–170	**171**–174	175–180	181+
<141	141–153	154–160	161–171	**172**–175	176–181	182+
<142	142–154	155–161	162–172	**173**–176	177–182	183+
<143	143–155	156–162	163–173	**174**–177	178–183	184+
<144	144–156	157–163	164–174	**175**–178	179–184	185+
<145	145–157	158–164	165–175	**176**–179	180–185	186+
<146	146–158	159–165	166–176	**177**–180	181–186	187+
<147	147–159	160–166	167–177	**178**–181	182–187	188+
<148	148–160	161–166	167–178	**179**–182	183–188	189+
<149	149–160	161–167	168–179	**180**–183	184–190	191+
<150	150–161	162–168	169–180	**181**–184	185–191	192+
<151	151–162	163–170	171–181	**182**–185	186–192	193+
<152	152–163	164–171	172–182	**183**–186	187–193	194+
<153	153–164	165–172	173–183	**184**–187	188–194	195+
<154	154–165	166–172	173–184	**185**–188	189–195	196+
<155	155–166	167–173	174–185	**186**–189	190–196	197+
<156	156–167	168–174	175–186	**187**–190	191–197	198+
<157	157–168	169–175	176–187	**188**–191	192–198	199+
<158	158–169	170–176	177–188	**189**–192	193–199	200+
<159	159–170	171–177	178–189	**190**–193	194–200	201+
<160	160–170	171–178	179–190	**191**–194	195–201	202+
<161	161–171	172–178	179–191	**192**–195	196–202	203+
<162	162–172	173–179	180–192	**193**–196	197–203	204+
<163	163–173	174–180	181–193	**194**–197	198–204	205+
<164	164–174	175–181	182–194	**195**–198	199–205	206

RUNNING & CROSS-COUNTRY SKIING HEART RATE ZONES

Find your LT heart rate (bold) in the "Zone 5a" column. Read across, left and right, for training zones.

ZONE 1: Active Recovery   **ZONE 2:** Aerobic Threshold   **ZONE 3:** Tempo   **ZONE 4:** Sub-Lactate Threshold
ZONE 5A: Lactate Threshold   **ZONE 5B:** Aerobic Capacity   **ZONE 5C:** Anaerobic Capacity

ZONE 1	ZONE 2	ZONE 3	ZONE 4	ZONE 5A	ZONE 5B	ZONE 5C
<120	120–126	127–133	134–139	**140–143**	144–149	150+
<120	120–127	128–134	135–140	**141–144**	145–150	151+
<121	121–129	130–135	136–141	**142–145**	146–151	152+
<122	122–130	131–136	137–142	**143–146**	147–152	153+
<123	123–131	132–137	138–143	**144–147**	148–153	154+
<124	124–132	133–138	139–144	**145–148**	149–154	155+
<125	125–133	134–139	140–145	**146–149**	150–155	156+
<125	125–134	135–140	141–146	**147–150**	151–156	157+
<126	126–135	136–141	142–147	**148**–151	152–157	158+
<127	127–135	136–142	143–148	**149**–152	153–158	159+
<128	128–136	137–143	144–149	**150**–153	154–158	159+
<129	129–137	138–144	145–150	**151**–154	155–159	160+
<130	130–138	139–145	146–151	**152**–155	156–160	161+
<131	131–139	140–146	147–152	**153**–156	157–161	162+
<132	132–140	141–147	148–153	**154**–157	158–162	163+
<132	132–141	142–148	149–154	**155**–158	159–164	165+
<133	133–142	143–149	150–155	**156**–159	160–165	166+
<134	134–143	144–150	151–156	**157**–160	161–166	167+
<135	135–143	144–151	152–157	**158**–161	162–167	168+
<136	136–144	145–152	153–158	**159**–162	163–168	169+
<137	137–145	146–153	154–159	**160**–163	164–169	170+
<137	137–146	147–154	155–160	**161**–164	165–170	171+
<138	138–147	148–155	156–161	**162**–165	166–171	172+
<139	139–148	149–155	156–162	**163**–166	167–172	173+
<140	140–149	150–156	157–163	**164**–167	168–174	175+
<141	141–150	151–157	158–164	**165**–168	169–175	176+
<142	142–151	152–158	159–165	**166**–169	170–176	177+
<142	142–152	153–159	160–166	**167**–170	171–177	178+

ZONE 1	ZONE 2	ZONE 3	ZONE 4	ZONE 5A	ZONE 5B	ZONE 5C
<143	143–153	154–160	161–167	**168**–171	172–178	179+
<144	144–154	155–161	162–168	**169**–172	173–179	180+
<145	145–155	156–162	163–169	**170**–173	174–179	180+
<146	146–156	157–163	164–170	**171**–174	175–180	181+
<146	146–156	157–164	165–171	**172**–175	176–182	183+
<147	147–157	158–165	166–172	**173**–176	177–183	184+
<148	148–157	158–166	167–173	**174**–177	178–184	185+
<149	149–158	159–167	168–174	**175**–178	179–185	186+
<150	150–159	160–168	169–175	**176**–179	180–186	187+
<151	151–160	161–169	170–176	**177**–180	181–187	188+
<152	152–161	162–170	171–177	**178**–181	182–188	189+
<153	153–162	163–171	172–178	**179**–182	183–189	190+
<154	154–163	164–172	173–179	**180**–183	184–190	191+
<155	155–164	165–173	174–180	**181**–184	185–192	193+
<155	155–165	166–174	175–181	**182**–185	186–193	194+
<156	156–166	167–175	176–182	**183**–186	187–194	195+
<157	157–167	168–176	177–183	**184**–187	188–195	196+
<158	158–168	169–177	178–184	**185**–188	189–196	197+
<159	159–169	170–178	179–185	**186**–189	190–197	198+
<160	160–170	171–179	180–186	**187**–190	191–198	199+
<160	160–170	171–179	180–187	**188**–191	192–199	200+
<161	161–171	172–180	181–188	**189**–192	193–200	201+
<162	162–172	173–181	182–189	**190**–193	194–201	202+
<163	163–173	174–182	183–190	**191**–194	195–201	202+
<164	164–174	175–183	184–191	**192**–195	196–202	203+
<165	165–175	176–184	185–192	**193**–196	197–203	204+
<166	166–176	177–185	186–193	**194**–197	198–204	205+
<166	166–177	178–186	187–194	**195**–198	199–205	206+
<167	167–178	179–187	188–195	**196**–199	200–206	207+
<168	168–178	179–188	189–196	**197**–198	199–207	208+
<169	169–179	180–189	190–197	**198**–201	202–208	209+
<170	170–180	181–190	191–198	**199**–202	203–209	210+
<171	171–181	182–191	192–199	**200**–203	204–210	211

SWIMMING HEART RATE ZONES

Find your LT heart rate (bold) in the "Zone 5a" column. Read across, left and right, for training zones.

ZONE 1: Active Recovery   ZONE 2: Aerobic Threshold   ZONE 3: Tempo   ZONE 4: Sub-Lactate Threshold
ZONE 5A: Lactate Threshold   ZONE 5B: Aerobic Capacity   ZONE 5C: Anaerobic Capacity

ZONE 1	ZONE 2	ZONE 3	ZONE 4	ZONE 5A	ZONE 5B	ZONE 5C
<101	101–114	115–122	123–129	**130**–133	134–135	136+
<102	102–115	116–122	123–130	**131**–134	135–138	139+
<102	102–116	117–123	124–131	**132**–135	136–140	141+
<103	103–117	118–124	125–132	**133**–136	137–141	142+
<104	104–118	119–125	126–133	**134**–137	138–142	143+
<105	105–118	119–126	127–134	**135**–138	139–143	144+
<105	105–119	120–127	128–135	**136**–139	140–144	145+
<106	106–120	121–128	129–136	**137**–140	141–145	146+
<107	107–121	122–129	130–137	**138**–141	142–146	147+
<108	108–122	123–130	131–138	**139**–142	143–147	148+
<109	109–123	124–131	132–139	**140**–143	144–148	149+
<109	109–124	125–132	133–140	**141**–144	145–149	150+
<110	110–125	126–133	134–141	**142**–145	146–150	151+
<111	111–125	126–134	135–142	**143**–146	147–151	152+
<112	112–126	127–135	136–143	**144**–147	148–152	153+
<112	112–127	128–136	137–144	**145**–148	149–153	154+
<113	113–128	129–137	138–145	**146**–149	150–154	155+
<114	114–129	130–138	139–146	**147**–150	151–155	156+
<115	115–130	131–138	139–147	**148**–151	152–156	157+
<116	116–131	132–139	140–148	**149**–152	153–157	158+
<116	116–132	133–140	141–149	**150**–153	154–158	159+
<117	117–133	134–141	142–150	**151**–154	155–159	160+
<118	118–133	134–142	143–151	**152**–155	156–160	161+
<119	119–134	135–143	144–152	**153**–156	157–161	162+
<119	119–135	136–144	145–153	**154**–157	158–162	163+
<120	120–136	137–145	146–154	**155**–158	159–163	164+
<121	121–137	138–146	147–155	**156**–159	160–164	165+
<122	122–138	139–147	148–156	**157**–160	161–165	166+

ZONE 1	ZONE 2	ZONE 3	ZONE 4	ZONE 5A	ZONE 5B	ZONE 5C
<123	123–139	140–148	149–157	**158**–161	162–166	167+
<123	123–140	141–149	150–158	**159**–162	163–167	168+
<124	124–141	142–150	151–159	**160**–163	164–168	169+
<125	125–141	142–151	152–160	**161**–164	165–169	170+
<126	126–142	143–152	153–161	**162**–165	166–170	171+
<126	126–143	144–153	154–162	**163**–166	167–171	172+
<127	127–144	145–154	155–163	**164**–167	168–172	173+
<128	128–145	146–154	155–164	**165**–168	169–173	174+
<129	129–146	147–155	156–165	**166**–169	170–174	175+
<130	130–147	148–156	157–166	**167**–170	171–175	176+
<130	130–148	149–157	158–167	**168**–171	172–176	177+
<131	131–148	149–158	159–168	**169**–172	173–177	178+
<132	132–149	150–159	160–169	**170**–173	174–178	179+
<133	133–150	151–160	161–170	**171**–174	175–179	180+
<133	133–151	152–161	162–171	**172**–175	176–180	181+
<134	134–152	153–162	163–172	**173**–176	177–181	182+
<135	135–153	154–163	164–173	**174**–177	178–182	183+
<136	136–154	155–164	165–174	**175**–178	179–183	184+
<137	137–155	156–165	166–175	**176**–179	180–184	185+
<137	137–156	157–166	167–176	**177**–180	181–185	186+
<138	138–156	157–167	168–177	**178**–181	182–186	187+
<139	139–157	158–168	169–178	**179**–182	183–187	188+
<140	140–158	159–169	170–179	**180**–183	184–188	189+
<140	140–159	160–170	171–180	**181**–184	185–189	190+
<141	141–160	161–171	172–181	**182**–185	186–190	191+
<142	142–161	162–171	172–182	**183**–186	187–191	192+
<143	143–162	163–172	173–183	**184**–187	188–192	193+
<143	144–163	164–173	174–184	**185**–188	189–193	194+
<144	144–164	165–174	175–185	**186**–189	190–194	195+
<145	145–164	165–175	176–186	**187**–190	191–195	196+
<146	146–165	166–176	177–187	**188**–191	192–196	197+
<147	147–166	167–177	178–188	**189**–192	193–197	198+
<147	147–167	168–178	179–189	**190**–193	194–198	199+

APPENDIX 3

ANNUAL TRAINING PLAN

ATHLETE: _____

ANNUAL HOURS: _____

SEASON GOALS:

_____
_____
_____
_____
_____

TRAINING OBJECTIVES:

_____
_____
_____
_____
_____
_____
_____

W - Weights
E - Endurance
F - Force
S - Speed Skill
M - Muscular Endurance
A - Anaerobic Endurance
P - Power
T - Weights

WK#	MONDAY	RACES	PRI	PERIOD	HOURS	COMMENTS	W	E	F	S	M	A	P	T
1														
2														
3														
4														
5														
6														
7														
8														
9														
10														
11														
12														
13														
14														
15														
16														
17														
18														
19														
20														
21														

WK#	MONDAY	RACES	PRI	PERIOD	HOURS	COMMENTS	W	E	F	S	M	A	P	T
22														
23														
24														
25														
26														
27														
28														
29														
30														
31														
32														
33														
34														
35														
36														
37														
38														
39														
40														
41														
42														
43														
44														
45														
46														
47														
48														
49														
50														
51														
52														

ANNUAL TRAINING PLAN / triathlon

ATHLETE: _____

ANNUAL HOURS: _____

SEASON GOALS:
_____
_____
_____
_____
_____

TRAINING OBJECTIVES:
_____
_____
_____
_____
_____
_____
_____

W - Weights
E - Endurance
F - Force
S - Speed Skill
M - Muscular Endurance
A - Anaerobic Endurance
P - Power
T - Weights

WK#	MONDAY	RACES	PRI	PERIOD	HOURS	COMMENTS	SWIM (W E F S M A P T)	BIKE (W E F S M A P T)	RUN (W E F S M A P T)
1									
2									
3									
4									
5									
6									
7									
8									
9									
10									
11									
12									
13									
14									
15									
16									
17									
18									
19									
20									
21									

WK#	MONDAY	RACES	PRI	PERIOD	HOURS	COMMENTS	SWIM	BIKE	RUN
							W E F S M A P T	W E F S M A P T	W E F S M A P T
22									
23									
24									
25									
26									
27									
28									
29									
30									
31									
32									
33									
34									
35									
36									
37									
38									
39									
40									
41									
42									
43									
44									
45									
46									
47									
48									
49									
50									
51									
52									

SAMPLE **MICROCYCLES**

The following tables each represent a one-week microcycle intended to fit into a specific meso-cycle. They are categorized by both sport type ("Steady State" or "Variably Paced") and your experience level. "Beginner" refers to someone in the first two years of the sport. "Inter-mediate" means an athlete with some experi-ence but who still has a long way to go to achieve his or her potential. "Advanced" means a highly experienced athlete who is competitive within his or her race category.

"Workout Ability" rows. Within each table, daily workouts are suggested by Training Triad ability (see Chapter 6 for ability details) for strengths and limiters (see Chapter 9 for details on strengths and limiters). The letters in these rows are ability abbreviations:

E = Endurance

F = Force

S = Speed Skill

M = Muscular Endurance

A = Anaerobic Endurance

P = Power

T = Test.

On some days the workout is suggested (for example, "E1"). In these cases, select a specific workout from Appendix 5 from that suggested grouping (for example, "E1b").

"Workout Code" rows. Select a workout or workouts from the menu in Appendix 5 based on the "Workout Ability" row above. Write in the code for each workout in these spaces. List only one workout code each day from the Appendix 5 menu in the "Workout Code" row unless instructed to do otherwise by the "Special" row. Note that "combined workouts" are described in Chapter 5.

"Duration" rows. These refer to Table 9.6. The words "short," "medium," and "long" are comparative terms and refer to the relative length of workouts planned for each day. For example, a week that has 8 hours planned would have 7 workout days of 2.0, 1.5, 1.25, 1.25, 1.0, 1.0, and 0 hours, according to Table 9.6. In this case, the "short" days are 1.0, 1.0, and 0 hours. The "medium" days are 1.25 and 1.25 hours. The "long" days are 2.0 and 1.5 hours. If a table below calls for 3 medium days instead of 2, either move a 1.0 from short or the 1.5 from long according to what best fits the require-ments of the table.

For prebuilt training plans for triathlon, duathlon, running, road cycling, mountain biking, bicycle tours, and century rides, go to www.TotalHRT.com and click on "Training Plans." These plans follow the concepts described in this book.

Steady State Sports

Examples: Running, bicycle time trial, bicycle century rides, mountain biking, swimming, cross-country skiing, rowing, triathlon, and duathlon.

PREP MICROCYCLES

	Mon	Tue	Wed	Thu	Fri	Sat	Sun
Workout ability	F1	S1	E1	F1	E1	S1	E1
Workout Code							
Duration	Short	Medium	Long	Short	Medium	Medium	Long
Special	Good day for weights or day off		May be cross training	Good day for weights or day off	May be cross training		May be cross training

beginner

BASE MICROCYCLES

	Mon	Tue	Wed	Thu	Fri	Sat	Sun
Workout ability	E1 or F1a or day off	Limiter: E1, F1, or S1	M1–M2	Strength: E1, F1a, or S1	E1	Limiter: F2 or S2	E2
Base 1 Workout Code							
Base 2 Workout Code							
Base 3 Workout Code							
Duration	Short	Medium	Long	Short	Medium	Medium	Long
Special	Good day for weights or day off		Gradually increase M from Z3 to Z4 over 8 wks	Good day for weights	Recovery day. May be day off.		Progress from E2a to E2b over a 4–6 wk period

beginner

BUILD MICROCYCLES

	Mon	Tue	Wed	Thu	Fri	Sat	Sun
Workout ability	E1 or F1a or day off	Limiter: E2, F2, or S2	M2	Strength: E2, F2, or S2	E1 or off	M1	E2
Build 1 Workout Code							
Build 2 Workout Code							
Duration	Short	Medium	Medium	Medium	Short	Long	Long
Special	Good day for weights or day off			Recovery day			

beginner

E = Endurance   **F** = Force   **S** = Speed Skill   **M** = Muscular Endurance   **A** = Anaerobic Endurance   **P** = Power   **T** = Test

APPENDIX 4

PEAK MICROCYCLES (see Chapter 8 for details on the Peak microcycles)

	Mon	Tue	Wed	Thu	Fri	Sat	Sun
Workout ability	E1 or F1a or day off	S1	M4	E1	S1	M4	E1
Workout Code							
Duration	Short	Long	Medium	Short	Medium	Medium	Long
Special	Good day for weights or day off		Simulate a a portion of the race	Recovery day		Simulate a a portion of the race	

RACE MICROCYCLES (A-Priority, Saturday Race)

	Mon	Tue	Wed	Thu	Fri	Sat	Sun
Workout ability	E1 or day off	E2	S1	E1 or day off	S3	Race	E1 or day off
Workout Code						Race	
Duration	0	Long	Medium	Short	Short	Varies	
Special	Day off is usually best. No weights today.			Day off is usually best option			Day off is usually best option

RACE MICROCYCLES (A-Priority, Sunday Race)

	Mon	Tue	Wed	Thu	Fri	Sat	Sun
Workout ability	E1 or day off	E2	S2	S1	E1 or day off	S3	Race
Workout Code							Race
Duration	Short	Long	Medium	Medium	Short	Short	Varies
Special	Day off is usually best. No weights today.				Day off is usually best option		

ALL REST AND RECOVERY (R&R) MICROCYCLES

	Mon	Tue	Wed	Thu	Fri	Sat	Sun
Workout ability	Day off, E1, or F1a	E1	E1 or S1	E1 or S1	T	Limiter: M1 or E2	Strength: M1 or E2
Workout Code							
Duration	Short	Short	Short	Medium	Medium	Long	Long
Special	Day off is usually best option				It is best that the test you use is repeated with each R&R week		

PREP MICROCYCLES

intermediate		Mon	Tue	Wed	Thu	Fri	Sat	Sun
	Workout ability	E1 or F1a or day off	S1	E1	F	E1	S1	E1
	Workout Code							
	Duration	Short	Medium	Long	Short	Medium	Medium	Long
	Special	Good day for weights or day off		May cross train	Good day for weights	May cross train		May cross train

BASE MICROCYCLES

intermediate		Mon	Tue	Wed	Thu	Fri	Sat	Sun
	Workout ability	E1 or F1a or day off	Limiter: E2, F2, or S2	M1, M2, or M3	Strength: E2, F2, S2, or weights	E1	Limiter: E2 or F2	Strength: E2 or F2
	Base 1 Workout Code							
	Base 2 Workout Code							
	Base 3 Workout Code							
	Duration	Short	Medium	Long	Medium	Short	Medium	Long
	Special	Good day for weights or day off		Gradually increase M from Z3 to Z5a over 8 wks	Good day for weights	Recovery day		Progress from E2a to E2b over a 4–6 wk period

BUILD MICROCYCLES

intermediate		Mon	Tue	Wed	Thu	Fri	Sat	Sun
	Workout ability	E1 or F1a or day off	Limiter: M1, M2, M3, and/or E2	Maintain: E2, F, and/or S2	Strength: M1, M2, M3, and/or A	E1	Limiter: M3 and/or E2	Strength: M3 and/or A
	Build1 Workout Code							
	Build 2 Workout Code							
	Duration	Short	Medium	Long	Medium	Short	Medium	Long
	Special	Good day for weights or day off	May combine 2 abilities in one workout	May combine 2 abilities in one workout. Change ability each week.	If weekend B race, reduce duration 50%. May combine M or A with E or F.	Recovery day. If weekend B race, reduce duration 50%.	May be race. If Sun B race, reduce duration 50%. May combine 2 abilities in 1 workout.	May combine 2 abilities in 1 workout. May be race. If Sat race, E or S only.

E = Endurance   **F** = Force   **S** = Speed Skill   **M** = Muscular Endurance   **A** = Anaerobic Endurance   **P** = Power   **T** = Test

APPENDIX 4

PEAK MICROCYCLES (see Chapter 8 for details on the Peak microcycles)

	Mon	Tue	Wed	Thu	Fri	Sat	Sun
Workout ability	F1a, S1, or day off	S2	M4 or A4	E1	S2	M4 or A4	E1
Workout Code							
Duration	Short	Medium	Long	Short	Medium	Long	Medium
Special	Good day for weights or day off		Simulate a portion of the race	Recovery day		May be race. If Sun B race, reduce duration 50%.	May be race. If Sat race, E only or day off.

intermediate

RACE MICROCYCLES (A-Priority, Saturday Race)

	Mon	Tue	Wed	Thu	Fri	Sat	Sun
Workout ability	E1 or day off	M4 or A4	M4 or A4	E1 or day off	S3	Race	E1 or day off
Workout Code						Race	
Duration	Short	Long	Medium	Short	Short	Varies	Medium
Special	Day off		Just a few reps at race-specific intensity	Rest day		Duration based on race	

intermediate

RACE MICROCYCLES (A-Priority, Sunday Race)

	Mon	Tue	Wed	Thu	Fri	Sat	Sun
Workout ability	E1 or day off	M4 or A4	M4 or A4	M4 or A4	E1 or day off	S3	Race
Workout Code							Race
Duration	Short	Long	Medium	Short	Short	Short	Varies
Special	Day off						Duration based on race

intermediate

ALL REST AND RECOVERY (R&R) MICROCYCLES

intermediate

	Mon	Tue	Wed	Thu	Fri	Sat	Sun
Workout ability	Day off, E1, or F1a	E1	E1 or S1	E1 or S1	T	Limiter: M1 or E2	Strength: M1 or E2
Workout Code							
Duration	Short	Short	Short	Medium	Medium	Long	Long
Special	Day off is usually best option				It is best that the test you use is repeated with each R&R week		

PREP MICROCYCLES

advanced

	Mon	Tue	Wed	Thu	Fri	Sat	Sun
Workout ability	E1, F1a, or day off	S1	E1	F1a or F2	E1	S1	E1
Workout Code							
Duration	Short	Medium	Long	Medium	Short	Medium	Long
Special	Good day for 1st weight workout of week		May be cross training	Good day for 2nd weight workout	May be cross training		May be cross training

BASE MICROCYCLES

advanced

	Mon	Tue	Wed	Thu	Fri	Sat	Sun
Workout ability	E1 or F1a or day off	Limiter: E2, F2, or S2	M1, M2, or M3	Strength: E2, F1a, F2, or S2	E1	Limiter: E2, F2, or S2	Strength: E2, F2, or S2
Base 1 Workout Code							
Base 2 Workout Code							
Base 3 Workout Code							
Duration	Short	Medium	Long	Medium	Short	Medium	Long
Special		May be 2–3 workouts	May be 2–3 workouts. Gradually increase M from Z3 to Z5a over 8 wks.	Good day for weights. May be 2–3 workouts.	Recovery day	May be 2–3 workouts	May be 2–3 workouts

APPENDIX 4

E = Endurance   **F** = Force   **S** = Speed Skill   **M** = Muscular Endurance   **A** = Anaerobic Endurance   **P** = Power   **T** = Test

BUILD MICROCYCLES

	Mon	Tue	Wed	Thu	Fri	Sat	Sun
Workout ability	E1, F1a, or day off	Limiter: M1, M2, M3, and/or A	Maintain: E2, F2b, and/or S2	Strength: M3 and/or A	E1	Limiter: M1, M2, M3, or A	Strength: M1, M2, M3, or A
Build 1 Workout Code							
Build 2 Workout Code							
Duration	Short	Medium	Long	Medium	Short	Long	Long
Special		May be 2 workouts. 2nd workout may be E1. In Build 2 combine M and A in a single workout.	May be 2 workouts. May combine 2 abilities in 1 workout. Train a different ability each week.	May be 2 workouts. 2nd workout may be E1. In Build 2 combine M and A in a single workout. If weekend B race, reduce duration 50% today.	Recovery day. If weekend B race, reduce duration 50% today.	May be 2 workouts. May combine 2 abilities in 1 workout. May be race. If Sun B race, reduce duration 50% today.	May be 2 workouts. May combine 2 abilities in 1 workout. May be race. If Sat race, E and/or S only today.

PEAK MICROCYCLES (see Chapter 8 for details on the Peak microcycles)

	Mon	Tue	Wed	Thu	Fri	Sat	Sun
Workout ability	E1, F1a, or day off	S2	M4 and/or A4	E1	S1	M4 and/or A4	E
Workout Code							
Duration	Short	Medium	Long	Short	Medium	Medium	Long
Special		May be 2 workouts	May be 2 workouts. Simulation should focus on intensity.	Recovery day	May be 2 workouts	May be 2 workouts. Simulation should focus on intensity. May be race. If Sun B race, reduce duration 50% today.	May be 2 workouts. May be race. If Sat was a race, E1 only today.

RACE MICROCYCLES (A-Priority, Saturday Race)

	Mon	Tue	Wed	Thu	Fri	Sat	Sun
Workout ability	E1 or day off	M4 or A4	M4 or A4	E1 or day off	S3	Race	E1 or day off
Workout Code						Race	
Duration	Short	Long	Medium	Short	Short	Varies	Medium
Special	Day off	May be 2 workouts with E1 or S1 as second	Just a few reps at race-specific intensity. May be 2 workouts with E1 or S1 as 2nd.	Rest day		Duration based on race	

APPENDIX 4

advanced

RACE MICROCYCLES (A-Priority, Sunday Race)

	Mon	Tue	Wed	Thu	Fri	Sat	Sun
Workout ability	E1 or day off	M4 or A4	M4 or A4	M4 or A4	E1 or day off	S3	Race
Workout Code							Race
Duration	**Short**	**Long**	**Medium**	**Short**	**Short**	**Short**	**Varies**
Special	Day off	May be 2 workouts with E1 or S1 as second	May be 2 workouts with E1 or S1 as second	Just a few reps at race-specific intensity. May be 2 workouts with E1 or S1 as second.			Duration on race

advanced

ALL REST AND RECOVERY (R&R) MICROCYCLES

	Mon	Tue	Wed	Thu	Fri	Sat	Sun
Workout ability	Day off, E1, or F1a	E1	E1 or S1	E1 or S1	T	Limiter: M1 or E2	Strength: M1 or E2
Workout Code							
Duration	**Short**	**Short**	**Short**	**Medium**	**Medium**	**Long**	**Long**
Special	Day off is usually best option				It is best that the test you use is repeated with each R&R week	May be 2 workouts with E1 as second	May be 2 workouts with E1 as second

advanced

Variably Paced Sports

Example: Bicycle road races, bicycle criteriums.

PREP MICROCYCLES

	Mon	Tue	Wed	Thu	Fri	Sat	Sun
Workout ability	F1a or F2	S1	E1	F1a or F2	E1	S1	E1
Workout Code							
Duration	**Short**	**Medium**	**Long**	**Short**	**Medium**	**Medium**	**Long**
Special	Good day for 1st weight workout of week		May be cross training	Good day for 2nd weight workout of week	May be cross training		May be cross training

beginner

E = Endurance   **F** = Force   **S** = Speed Skill   **M** = Muscular Endurance   **A** = Anaerobic Endurance   **P** = Power   **T** = Test

BASE MICROCYCLES

	Mon	Tue	Wed	Thu	Fri	Sat	Sun
Workout ability	E1, F1a, or day off	Limiter: E1, F2, or S1	M1 or M2	Strength: E1, F2 ,or S1	E1	Limiter: F2 or P1	E2
Base 1 Workout Code							
Base 2 Workout Code							
Base 3 Workout Code							
Duration	Short	Medium	Long	Short	Medium	Medium	Long
Special	Good day for 1st weight workout of week		Gradually increase M from Z3 to Z4 over 8 wks	Good day for 2nd weight workout of week	Recovery day. May be day off.		

BUILD MICROCYCLES

	Mon	Tue	Wed	Thu	Fri	Sat	Sun
Workout ability	E1, F1a, or day off	Limiter: E2, F2b, or S2	M2	Strength: E2, F2b, or P1	E1 or off	M1	E2
Build 1 Workout Code							
Build 2 Workout Code							
Duration	Short	Medium	Medium	Medium	Short	Long	Long
Special	Good day for weights or day off				Recovery day		

PEAK MICROCYCLES (see Chapter 8 for details on the Peak microcycles)

	Mon	Tue	Wed	Thu	Fri	Sat	Sun
Workout ability	E1, F1a, or day off	S1	M3, M4, or A3	E1	S1	M3, M4, or A3	E1
Workout Code							
Duration	Short	Long	Medium	Short	Medium	Medium	Long
Special	Good day for weights or day off		Simulate a portion of the race.	Recovery day		Simulate a portion of the race	

RACE MICROCYCLES (A-Priority, Saturday Race)

	Mon	Tue	Wed	Thu	Fri	Sat	Sun
Workout ability	E1 or day off	E2	P1	E1 or day off	S3	Race	E1 or day off
Workout Code						Race	
Duration	0	Long	Medium	Short	Short	Varies	
Special	Day off is usually best. No weights.			Day off is usually best option			Day off is usually best option

APPENDIX 4

beginner

RACE MICROCYCLES (A-Priority, Sunday Race)

beginner		Mon	Tue	Wed	Thu	Fri	Sat	Sun
	Workout ability	E1 or day off	E2	P1	S1	E1 or day off	S3	Race
	Workout Code							Race
	Duration	Short	Long	Medium	Medium	Short	Short	Varies
	Special	Day off is usually best. No weights.				Day off is usually best option		

ALL REST AND RECOVERY (R&R) MICROCYCLES

beginner		Mon	Tue	Wed	Thu	Fri	Sat	Sun
	Workout ability	E1, F1a, or day off	E1	E1 or S1	E1 or S1	T	Limiter: M1 or E2	Strength: M1 or E2
	Workout Code							
	Duration	Short	Short	Short	Medium	Medium	Long	Long
	Special	Day off is usually best option			It is best that the test you use is repeated with each R&R week			

PREP MICROCYCLES

intermediate		Mon	Tue	Wed	Thu	Fri	Sat	Sun
	Workout ability	E1, F1a, or day off	S1	E1	F1a or F2a	E1	S1	E1
	Workout Code							
	Duration	Short	Medium	Long	Short	Medium	Medium	Long
	Special	Good day for 1st weight workout of week		May cross train	Good day for 2nd weight workout of week	May cross train		May cross train

BASE MICROCYCLES

intermediate		Mon	Tue	Wed	Thu	Fri	Sat	Sun
	Workout ability	E1, F1a, or day off	Limiter: E2, F2, or P1	M1, M2, or M3	Strength: E2, F1a, F2b, or S2	E1	Limiter: E2 or F2	Strength: E2 or F2
	Base 1 Workout Code							
	Base 2 Workout Code							
	Base 3 Workout Code							
	Duration	Short	Medium	Long	Medium	Short	Medium	Long
	Special	Good day for 1st weight workout of week		Gradually increase M from Z3 to Z5 over 8 wks. No group ride until Base 3.	Good day for 2nd weight workout of week	Recovery day		

E = Endurance   **F** = Force   **S** = Speed Skill   **M** = Muscular Endurance   **A** = Anaerobic Endurance   **P** = Power   **T** = Test

APPENDIX 4

BUILD MICROCYCLES

	Mon	Tue	Wed	Thu	Fri	Sat	Sun
Workout ability	E1, F1a, or day off	Limiter: M1, M2, M3, P2, and/or E2	Maintain: E2, F2b, and/or S2	Strength: M1, M2, M3, P2, and/or A	E1	Limiter: M3, A3, and/or E2	Strength: M3 or A3
Build 1 Workout Code							
Build 2 Workout Code							
Duration	Short	Medium	Long	Medium	Short	Medium	Long
Special	Good day for weights or day off	May combine 2 abilities in 1 workout	May combine 2 abilities in 1 workout. Change ability each week.	If weekend B race, reduce duration 50%. May combine M or A with E or F.	Recovery day. If weekend B race, reduce duration 50%.	May be race. If Sun B race, reduce duration 50%. May combine 2 abilities in 1 workout.	May combine 2 abilities in 1 workout. May be race. If Sat race, E or S only.

intermediate

PEAK MICROCYCLES (see Chapter 8 for details on the Peak microcycles)

	Mon	Tue	Wed	Thu	Fri	Sat	Sun
Workout ability	F1a, S1, or day off	S2	P3, M3, M4, A3, or A4	E1	S2	P3, M3, M4, A3, or A4	E1
Workout Code							
Duration	Short	Medium	Long	Short	Medium	Long	Medium
Special	Good day for weights or day off		Simulate a portion of the race. Simulation should focus on intensity.	Recovery day		Race simulation. May be race. If Sun B race, reduce duration 50%.	May be race. If Sat race, E only or day off.

intermediate

RACE MICROCYCLES (A-Priority, Saturday Race)

	Mon	Tue	Wed	Thu	Fri	Sat	Sun
Workout ability	E1 or day off	P3, M3, M4, A3, or A4	M4 or A4	E1 or day off	S3	Race	E1 or day off
Workout Code						Race	
Duration	Short	Long	Medium	Short	Short	Varies	Medium
Special	Rest day		Just a few reps at race-specific intensity	Rest day		Duration based on race	

intermediate

RACE MICROCYCLES (A-Priority, Sunday Race)

	Mon	Tue	Wed	Thu	Fri	Sat	Sun
Workout ability	E1 or day off	P3, M3, M4, A3, or A4	P3, M3, M4, A3, or A4	M4 or A4	E1 or day off	S3	Race
Workout Code							Race
Duration	Short	Long	Medium	Short	Short	Short	Varies
Special	Rest day	Group workout today or tomorrow, but not both		Just a few reps at race-specific intensity			Duration based on race

intermediate

ALL REST AND RECOVERY (R&R) MICROCYCLES

	Mon	Tue	Wed	Thu	Fri	Sat	Sun
Workout ability	Day off, E1, or F1a	E1	E1 or S1	E1 or S1	T	Limiter: M3 A3, and/or E2	Strength: M3 or A3
Workout Code							
Duration	Short	Short	Short	Medium	Medium	Medium	Long
Special	Day off is usually best option				It is best that the test you use is repeated with each R&R week	May be race. If Sun B race, reduce duration 50%. May combine 2 abilities in 1 workout.	May be race. If Sat race, E or S only today.

intermediate

PREP MICROCYCLES

	Mon	Tue	Wed	Thu	Fri	Sat	Sun
Workout ability	E1, F1a, or day off	S1	E1	F1a or F2a	E1	S1	E1
Workout Code							
Duration	Short	Medium	Long	Medium	Short	Medium	Long
Special	Good day for 1st weight workout of week			Good day for weights	Recovery day		

advanced

BASE MICROCYCLES

	Mon	Tue	Wed	Thu	Fri	Sat	Sun
Workout ability	E1, F1a, or day off	Limiter: E2, F2b, or P1	M1, M2, or M3	Strength: E2, F1a, F2b, S2, or weights	E1	Limiter: E2 or F2b	Strength: E2 or F2b
Base 1 Workout Code							
Base 2 Workout Code							
Base 3 Workout Code							
Duration	Short	Medium	Long	Medium	Short	Medium	Long
Special	Good day for weights or day off	May be 2–3 workouts	May be 2–3 workouts. Gradually increase M from Z3 to Z5a over 8 wks. No group ride until Base 3.	Good day for weights or day off. May be 2–3 workouts.	Recovery day	May be 2–3 workouts	May be 2–3 workouts

advanced

E = Endurance   **F** = Force   **S** = Speed Skill   **M** = Muscular Endurance   **A** = Anaerobic Endurance   **P** = Power   **T** = Test

APPENDIX 4

BUILD MICROCYCLES

	Mon	Tue	Wed	Thu	Fri	Sat	Sun
Workout ability	E1, F1a, or day off	Limiter: M1, M2, M3, P2, and/or E2	Maintain: E2, F2b, and/or S2	Strength: M1, M2, M3, P2, and/or A	E1	Limiter: M3, A3, and/or E2	Strength: M3 or A3
Build 1 Workout Code							
Build 2 Workout Code							
Duration	Short	Medium	Long	Medium	Short	Long	Long
Special	Good day for weights or day off	May be 2 workouts. 2nd workout may be E1. In Build 2 combine M and P in a single workout.	May be 2 workouts. May combine 2 abilities in 1 workout. Train a different ability each week.	May be 2 workouts. 2nd workout may be E1. In Build 2 combine M and A in a single workout If weekend B race, reduce duration 50% today.	Recovery day. If weekend B race, reduce duration 50% today.	May be 2 workouts. May combine 2 abilities in 1 workout. May be race. If Sun B race, reduce duration 50% today.	May be 2 workouts. May combine 2 abilities in 1 workout. May be race. If Sat race, E and/or S only today.

advanced

PEAK MICROCYCLES (see Chapter 8 for details on the Peak microcycles)

	Mon	Tue	Wed	Thu	Fri	Sat	Sun
Workout ability	F1a, S1, or day off	S2	P3, M3, M4, A3, or A4	E1	S2	P3, M3, M4, A3, or A4	E
Workout Code							
Duration	Short	Medium	Long	Short	Medium	Long	Medium
Special	Good day for weights or day off	May be 2 workouts	May be 2 workouts. Simulation should focus on intensity.	Recovery day	May be 2 workouts	May be 2 workouts. Simulation should focus on intensity. Race simulation. May be race. If Sun B race, reduce duration 50% today.	May be 2 workouts. May be race. If Sat was a race, E1 only today.

advanced

RACE MICROCYCLES (A-Priority, Saturday Race)

	Mon	Tue	Wed	Thu	Fri	Sat	Sun
Workout ability	E1 or day off	P3, M3, M4, A3, or A4	M4 or A4	E1 or day off	S3	Race	E1 or day off
Workout Code						Race	
Duration	Short	Long	Medium	Short	Short	Varies	Medium
Special	Rest day	May be 2 workouts with E1 or S1 as 2nd	Just a few reps at race-specific intensity. May be 2 workouts with E1 or S1 as 2nd.	Rest day		Duration based on race	

advanced

RACE MICROCYCLES (A-Priority, Sunday Race)

	Mon	Tue	Wed	Thu	Fri	Sat	Sun
Workout ability	E1 or day off	P3, M3, M4, A3, or A4	P3, M3, M4, A3, or A4	M4 or A4	E1 or day off	S3	Race
Workout Code							Race
Duration	**Short**	**Long**	**Medium**	**Short**	**Short**	**Short**	**Varies**
Special	Rest day	May be 2 workouts with E1 or S1 as second. Group workout either today or tomorrow but not both.	May be 2 workouts with E1 or S1 as second	Just a few reps at race-specific intensity. May be 2 workouts with E1 or S1 as second.			Duration based on race

(left margin: advanced)

ALL REST AND RECOVERY (R&R) MICROCYCLES

	Mon	Tue	Wed	Thu	Fri	Sat	Sun
Workout ability	E1 or F1a	E1	E1 or S1	E1 or S1	T	Limiter: M1, A3b or E2	Strength: M1, A3b, or E2
Workout Code							
Duration	**Short**	**Short**	**Short**	**Medium**	**Medium**	**Long**	**Long**
Special	Day off is usually best option				It is best that the test you use is repeated with each R&R week	May be 2 workouts with E1 as 2nd. May be race. If Sun B race, reduce duration 50%. May combine 2 abilities in 1 workout.	May be 2 workouts with E1 as 2nd. May be race. If Sat race, E or S only today.

(left margin: advanced)

(right margin: APPENDIX 4)

E = Endurance   **F** = Force   **S** = Speed Skill   **M** = Muscular Endurance   **A** = Anaerobic Endurance   **P** = Power   **T** = Test

SAMPLE **WORKOUTS**

The following are the workout codes referred to in Appendix 4. The abilities (endurance, force, speed skill, muscular endurance, anaerobic endurance, and power) are described in Chapter 6. The Test workouts at the end of this appendix are described in Chapter 4.

The suggested workouts that follow may be altered to better fit the demands of your sport. As an example, for swimming, the work intervals are better determined by pool length than by duration. And for swim interval workouts the rest intervals may be reduced considerably, perhaps by as much as 50 to 70 percent, because of more rapid recovery that occurs when standing in water. For cycling, cadence is often altered to change the nature of the stress. High cadences tend to have a greater effect on aerobic capacity, while lower cadences place more stress on the muscles.

For detailed guidance for swim workouts based on the Total Heart Rate Training Program, see the book *Workouts in a Binder for Swimmers, Triathletes, and Coaches,* by Nick Hansen and Eric Hansen. For indoor bicycle workouts similar to what is described here, look for *Workouts in a Binder for Indoor Cycling,* by Dirk Friel and Wes Hobson. These books are available at http://store.velogear.com.

For detailed workouts designed by experience level and event, go to www.TotalHRT.com and click on "Training Plans."

Endurance (E) Workouts

E1A RECOVERY

Stay in Zone 1 for the entire workout to allow for recovery from previous, more stressful workout.

E1B RECOVERY CROSS TRAIN

In an endurance sport or activity other than your primary sport, exercise lightly in Zone 1. If you don't know the heart rate zones for this alternative sport, then use a 1 (extremely easy) to 10 (extremely hard) perceived exertion scale and exercise at below a level 4. This workout is especially recommended for runners.

E2A LOW AEROBIC THRESHOLD

Following warm-up, maintain a steady effort in the lower half of your Zone 2 for 1 to 4 hours. The exact duration depends on your sport and the targeted time for your next A- priority event. Runners and swimmers should aim for 1 to 2 hours. If the duration of your A race falls between 1 and 2 hours, swim or run in lower Zone 2 for that amount of time. If greater than 2 hours, then swim or run 2 hours in lower Zone 2. If less than 1 hour, then swim or run 1 hour in lower Zone 2. For all other sports, the range is 2 to 4 hours, using the same method to determine workout duration as for running and swimming.

E2B HIGH AEROBIC THRESHOLD

This workout is exactly the same as E2a, except that you should use the upper half of your Zone 2. E2a should be done several times before progressing to E2b.

Force (F) Workouts

F1A WEIGHT TRAINING

Lift weights, using exercises that closely mimic the movements of your sport.

F2A CROSS TRAIN FORCE

Use an activity or sport other than your primary sport. Create a moderate amount of resistance in some way and vary heart rate from Zone 1 to Zone 3 throughout the exercise session. For example, fill a backpack with books and hike on hilly terrain. Or ride a bicycle in a high gear so that you pedal with a low cadence.

F2B SPORT-SPECIFIC FORCE

In your primary sport, warm up and then exercise with some sort of resistance such as hilly terrain, wind, rough water, tethers, or drag devices. Emphasize muscular activity to overcome the resistance. This often means using a lower cadence than usual. Heart rate should rise and fall throughout the session, going no higher than Zone 4.

Speed Skill (S) Workouts

S1A BASIC SKILLS

Using basic drills appropriate for your event, work on fundamental, sport-specific skills, especially those that need improvement. The drills should be done in an exaggerated manner at a slow rhythm.

S2A ADVANCED SKILLS

Work on your sport's more advanced skills at a cadence or rhythm that is appropriate for your sport. For example, swimmers typically use a cadence of 45 to 55 cycles per minute, cyclists 80 to 100, and runners 85 to 95. These skills may include sprinting form for variably paced events such as bicycle road racing.

S3A WARM-UP SKILL

Rehearse the warm-up you will do before your next A-priority race. The warm-up should include several seconds to several minutes at your goal race heart rate.

Muscular Endurance (M) Workouts

M1A TEMPO INTERVALS

Warm up and then complete 30 to 90 minutes of work intervals in Zone 3. The work intervals are 12 to 20 minutes long with recovery intervals that are one-fourth as long (for example, following a 12-minute work interval, recover for 3 minutes). Gradually increase the amount of Zone 3 training time in this workout over the Base 1 and Base 2 periods.

M1B STEADY TEMPO

Following warm-up, train steadily for 20 to 90 minutes in Zone 3. Slowly build from 20 minutes to a longer duration over several weeks.

M2A CRUISE INTERVALS

Warm up, raising your heart rate from Zone 1 to Zone 3 by varying the effort. Then complete a total of 30 to 60 minutes of work intervals that are 6 to 2 minutes long. The recovery intervals are one-fourth the duration of the preceding work interval (for example, following a 6-minute work interval, recover for 90 seconds). When first doing cruise intervals, the work interval durations may descend (such as 12, 10, 8, 6 minutes) to allow for gradual adaptation to longer times at this intensity. End this workout with a short cool-down in Zone 1.

M2B CRUISE STEADY STATE

Warm up, raising your heart rate from Zone 1 to Zone 3 by varying the effort. Train steadily in Zone 4 for 20 to 30 minutes. This is an advanced workout that is best done following the establishment of good Zone 4 fitness with cruise intervals. End this workout with a short cool-down in Zone 1.

M3A THRESHOLD CRUISE INTERVALS

These are the same as M2a cruise intervals except the intensity builds into Zone 5a as the work interval progresses.

M3B THRESHOLD CRUISE STEADY STATE

This is done the same as M2b cruise steady state, but the heart rate and intensity are allowed to increase into Zone 5a in the latter minutes of each work interval.

M4A SHORT RACE SIMULATION (STEADY STATE EVENTS)

Warm up well by raising your heart rate to Zone 3 before starting the mainset. Then simulate a small portion of your next A-priority, steady state event with an emphasis on the proper heart rate zone intensity. You may consider using this workout to simulate pacing at various times in the event, goal power levels, terrain, race equipment and clothing, weather conditions such as heat and humidity, race strategy or tactics, and refueling plans. Consider focusing especially on portions of the race plan about which you are unsure.

M4B LONG RACE SIMULATION (STEADY STATE EVENTS)

This workout is the same as M4a except it is longer and focuses on a bigger portion of the A-priority event. The simulation portion of the workout could be as long as half the targeted duration of your event.

M4C CRISS-CROSS

Warm up, raising your heart rate from Zone 1 to Zone 3 by varying the effort. Then exercise continuously for 12 to 30 minutes by allowing heart rate to rise and fall between lower Zone 4 and Zone 5a, as you feel like doing. This is essentially a free-form workout done around the lactate threshold. End this workout with a short cool-down in Zone 1.

Anaerobic Endurance (A) Workouts

A1A SHORT AEROBIC CAPACITY INTERVALS

Warm up by ratcheting your heart rate up from Zone 1 to Zone 4, varying the effort with an interval or fartlek format (see A3a Fartlek workout below). Then alternate 30 seconds at aerobic capacity effort (RPE 9), pace, or power (heart rate responds too slowly to be effective for gauging intensity in this workout). Recover for 30 seconds after each work interval. Build to about 24 such intervals over a 3- to 4-week period. Be conservative as far as effort on the first few intervals. If you fade in the last few intervals, you probably started out too fast. End this workout with a short cool-down in Zone 1.

A2A LONG AEROBIC CAPACITY INTERVALS

Warm up by ratcheting your heart rate up from Zone 1 to Zone 4, varying the effort with an interval or fartlek format. Immediately following the warm-up, complete 12 to 20 minutes total of work intervals that are each 2 to 4 minutes long. The recovery interval initially is as long as the preceding work interval. Over the course of several weeks the recovery intervals are slightly shortened to better simulate the event. As with all interval workouts, at the completion of this mainset you should feel like you could have done one more work interval. End this workout with a short cool-down in Zone 1.

A2B HYDROGEN STACKER

Warm up by ratcheting your heart rate up from Zone 1 to Zone 4, varying the effort with an interval or fartlek format. This is a very challenging workout that creates extremely high levels of acidosis. If you do short but fast endurance events such as bicycle criterium racing, however, this mainset will develop the capacity to remove and buffer the acid, allowing you to continue pushing the effort. Here is how it's done: Do 4, 20- to 40-second, near-maximum-effort (RPE 10) sprints with 20-second recovery intervals. That is 1 set. Do 1 to 3 such sets in a mainset with 5 minutes of very easy recovery (passive and active) between sets. The duration of the work intervals and the number of sets depends on the demands of the event for which you are training. Start at the low end of each and add duration and sets as your fitness improves. End this workout with a short cool-down in Zone 1. *Do not do this workout unless you are an experienced and very fit athlete with a low risk for cardiovascular disease.* It is extremely stressful. One of these in a week is plenty. Allow at least 3 days for recovery afterward.

A3A FARTLEK

This is mostly an unstructured workout done at all intensities. Warm up by gradually increasing the intensity of the workout and raising your heart rate to Zone 3. Then "play" with speed (in Swedish the word for speedplay is *fartlek*) by varying both the intensity and the duration of the high and low intensities. The intensity may be as high or low as you feel like going on a given day. The duration of the speedplay portions and how long the workout lasts is unstructured and done strictly based on how you feel on the day of the workout. End this workout with a short cool-down in Zone 1.

A3B GROUP WORKOUT

Do your workout with a group of training partners. In the Base period the intensity of this workout should stay below Zone 5a with a considerable amount of time accumulated in Zones 2, 3, and 4. Stay away from groups at this time of year that like to "hammer." Such training is counterproductive in the Base period. In the Build and Peak periods, use this workout to simulate race conditions and use appropriate heart rate zones based on your goal intensities for your next A-priority event.

A4A SHORT RACE SIMULATION (VARIABLY PACED EVENTS)

Warm up well by raising your heart rate to Zone 3 before starting the mainset. Then simulate a small portion of your next A-priority, steady state event with an emphasis on the proper heart rate zone intensity. You may consider using this workout to simulate pacing at various times in the event, goal power levels, terrain, race equipment and clothing, weather conditions such as heat and humidity, race strategy or tactics, and refueling plans. Consider focusing especially on portions of the race plan about which you are unsure. This may be a group workout.

A4B LONG RACE SIMULATION (VARIABLY PACED EVENTS)

This workout is the same as A4a except it is longer and focuses on a bigger portion of the

A-priority event. The simulation portion of the workout could be as long as half the targeted duration of your event. This also may be a group workout.

Power (P) Workouts

P1A CP INTERVALS

The purpose of this mainset is to improve your body's capacity for power development and to enhance its ability to recover by generating more creatine phosphate following sprints. Warm up by gradually increasing the intensity of the workout and raising your heart rate to Zone 3. Then once every 5 minutes of the mainset do a maximum-effort (RPE 10) for 8 to 15 seconds. Do not allow good form to be compromised. If you begin to get sloppy or if power or velocity fades, stop the mainset and begin the cool-down. Do as many as 15 of these in a mainset. You may break the intervals into sets of 3 to 5 work intervals each, with 10 minutes of recovery between sets. Again, do not continue if form begins to break down. End this workout with a short cool-down in Zone 1.

P2A POWER LACTATE INTERVALS

Warm up by gradually increasing the intensity of the workout and raising your heart rate to Zone 3. Then do 5, 20- to 40-second, maximum-effort (RPE 10) sprints with 3-minute recovery intervals. That is 1 set. Do 1 to 3 such sets in a mainset with 10 minutes of easy recovery between sets. The duration of the work intervals and the number of sets depends on the demands of the event for which you are training. Start at the low end of each and add duration and sets as your fitness improves. This workout improves your capacity to maintain a high level of power even though acid is flooding the muscles. The long recoveries are necessary to remove most of the acid so that power may be near maximum for each work interval. End this workout with a short cool-down in Zone 1.

P3A PARTNER SPRINTS

Do P2a with a training partner with a similar power ability.

Test (T) Workouts

T1A TEMPO TIME TRIAL

See the Tempo Time Trial sidebar in Chapter 4 for details.

T1B RAMP TEST

See the Ramp Test sidebar in Chapter 4 for details.

SUGGESTED READING

Burke E. (editor). 1998. *Precision Heart Rate Training*. Champaign, IL: Human Kinetics.

Friel D. and Hobson W. 2006. *Workouts in a Binder for Indoor Cycling*. Boulder, CO: VeloPress.

Friel J. 1996. *The Cyclist's Training Bible*. Boulder, CO: VeloPress.

Friel J. 1998. *The Triathlete's Training Bible*. Boulder, CO: VeloPress.

Friel J. 2000. *The Mountain Biker's Training Bible*. Boulder, CO: VeloPress.

Friel J. and Byrn G. 2003. *Going Long*. Boulder, CO: VeloPress.

Hansen N. and Hansen E. 2005. *Workouts in a Binder for Swimmers, Triathletes, and Coaches*. Boulder, CO: VeloPress.

Janssen PGJM. 1989. *Training, Lactate, Pulse Rate*. Polar Electro Oy.

BIBLIOGRAPHY

CHAPTER 1

Bell J.M. and Bassey E.J. 1996. Postexercise heart rates and pulse palpation as a means of determining exercising intensity in an aerobic dance class. *British Journal of Sports Medicine* 30 (1): 48–52.

Clapp III J. and Little K. 1994. The physiological response of instructors and participants to three aerobics regimens. *Medicine and Science in Sports and Exercise* 26 (8): 1041–46.

Karvonen J., Chwalbinska-Moneta J., and Säynäjäkangas S. 1984. Comparison of heart rates measured by ECG and microcomputer. *The Physician and Sportsmedicine* 12 (6): 65–69.

Leger L. and Thivierge M. 1988. Heart rate monitors: validity, stability and functionality. *The Physician and Sportsmedicine* 16 (5): 143–51.

Leger L. and Tokmakidis S. 1988. Use of the heart rate deflection point to assess the anaerobic threshold. *Journal of Applied Physiology* 64 (4): 1758–60.

Seaward B., Sleamaker R., McAuliffe T., and Clapp J. 1990. The precision and accuracy of a portable heart rate monitor. *Biomedical Instrumentation & Technology* 24 (1): 37–41.

Treffene R.J. 1975. An investigation of the ECG in sports and sports medicine using radiotelemetry. Master's thesis, University of London.

Vogelaere P., De Meyer F., Duquet W., and Vandevelde P. 1986. Vergleich zwischen "Sport Tester PE 3000" und Holter-EKG zur Messung der Herzfrequenz (Sport Tester PE 3000 vs Holter ECG for the measurement of heart frequency). *Science & Sports* 1 (4): 321–29.

CHAPTER 2

Achten J., Gleeson M., and Jeukendrup A.E. 2002. Determination of the exercise intensity that elicits maximal fat oxidation. *Medicine and Science in Sports and Exercise* 34 (1): 92–97.

Anderson O. 1994. What exercise intensity is best for breaking down fat? *Running Research News* 1 (10): 1, 4–10.

Boulay M.R., Simoneau J.A., and Bouchard C. 1997. Monitoring high-intensity endurance exercise with heart rate and thresholds. *Medicine and Science in Sports and Exercise* 29 (1): 125–32.

Cassady S. and Nielsen D.H. 1992. Cardiorespiratory responses of healthy subjects to calisthenics performed on land versus in water. *Physical Therapy* 72 (7): 532–37.

Cole C.R. et al. 1999. Heart-rate recovery immediately after exercise as a predictor of mortality. *New England Journal of Medicine* 341 (18): 1351–57.

Finn I.B., Iuvone P.M., and Holtzman S.G. 1990. Depletion of catecholamines in the brain of rats differentially affects stimulation of locomotor activity by caffeine, D-amphetamine, and methylphenidate. *Neuropharmacology* 29 (7): 625–31.

Fixx J.F. 1977. *The Complete Book of Running.* New York: Random House.

Gnehm P., Reichbach S., Altpeter E., Widmer H., and Hoppeler H. 1997. Influence of different racing positions on metabolic cost in elite cyclists. *Medicine and Science in Sports and Exercise* 29 (6):8, 18–23.

Gonzalez-Alonso J., Mora-Rodriguez R., and Coyle E.F. 2000. Stroke volume during exercise: interaction of environment and hydration. *American Journal of Physiology* 278: H321–30.

Hawkins S. and Wiswell R. 2003. Rate and mechanism of maximal oxygen consumption decline with aging: implications for exercise training. *Sports Medicine* 33 (12): 877–88

Heath G.W., Hagberg J.M., Ehsani A.A., and Holloszy J.O. 1981. A physiological comparison of young and older endurance athletes. *Journal of Applied Physiology* 51 (3): 634–40.

Hedelin R., Wiklund U., Bjerle P., and Henriksson-Larsen K. 2000. Short-term overtraining: effects on performance, circulatory responses, and heart rate variability. *Medicine and Science in Sports and Exercise* 32: 1480–84.

Jacobs I., Romet T.T., and Kerrigan-Brown D. 1985. Muscle glycogen depletion during exercise at 9 degrees C and 21 degrees C. *European Journal of Applied Physiology and Occupational Physiology* 54 (1): 35–39.

Kasch F.W., Boyer J.L., Van Camp S., Nettl F., Verity L.S., and Wallace J.P. 1995. Cardiovascular changes with age and exercise. A 28-year longitudinal study. *Scandinavian Journal of Medicine & Science in Sports* 5 (3): 147–51.

Kravitz L., Robergs R.A., Heyward V.H., Wagner D.R., and Powers K. 1997. Exercise mode and gender comparisons of energy expenditure at self-selected intensities. *Medicine and Science in Sports and Exercise* 29 (8): 1028–35.

Reilly T. and Garrett R. 1998. Investigation of diurnal variation in sustained exercise performance. *Ergonomics* 41 (8): 1085–94.

Robertson D., Frolich J.C., Carr R.K., Watson J.T., Hollifield J.W., Shand D.G., and Oates J.A. 1978. Effects of caffeine on plasma renin activity, catecholamines and blood pressure. *New England Journal of Medicine* 298 (4): 181–86.

Rogers M.A., Hagberg J.M., Martin W.H. 3rd, Ehsani A.A., and Holloszy J.O. 1990. Decline in VO_2 max with aging in master athletes and sedentary men. *Journal of Applied Physiology* 68 (5): 2195–99.

Sink K.R., Thomas T.R., Araujo J., and Hill S.F. 1989. Fat energy use and plasma lipid changes associated with exercise intensity and temperature. *European Journal of Applied Physiology and Occupational Physiology* 58 (5): 508–13.

Stevens G.H., Graham T.E., and Wilson B.A. 1987. Gender differences in cardiovascular and metabolic responses to cold and exercise. *Canadian Journal of Physiology and Pharmacology* 65 (2): 165-71.

Swine C. 1992. Aging of heart function in man. *La Presse Médicale* 22; 21 (26): 1216–21.

Tanaka H., Fukumoto S., Osaka Y., Ogawa S., Yamaguchi H., and Miyamoto H. 1991. Distinctive effects of three different modes of exercise on oxygen uptake, heart rate and blood lactate and pyruvate. *International Journal of Sports Medicine* 12: 433–38.

Tate C.A., Hyek M.F., and Taffet G.E. 1994. Mechanisms for the responses of cardiac muscle to physical activity in old age. *Medicine and Science in Sports and Exercise* 26 (5): 561–67.

Trappe S.W., Costill D.L., Vukovich M.D., Jones J., and Melham T. 1996. Aging among elite distance runners: a 22-year longitudinal study. *Journal of Applied Physiology* 80 (1): 285–90.

Tremblay A., Simoneau J.A., and Bouchard C. 1994. Impact of exercise intensity on body fatness and skeletal muscle metabolism. *Metabolism* 43 (7): 814–18.

CHAPTER 3

Boulay M.R., Simoneau J.A., and Bouchard C. 1997. Monitoring high-intensity endurance exercise with heart rate and thresholds. *Medicine and Science in Sports and Exercise* 29 (1): 125–32.

Cheng B., Kuipers H., Snyder A.C., et al. 1992. A new approach for the determination of ventilatory and lactate thresholds. *International Journal of Sports Medicine* 13 (7): 518–22.

Cooper K.H. et al. 1977. Age-fitness adjusted maximal heart rates. *Medicine and Science in Sports and Exercise* 10: 78–86.

DiCarlo L.J. et al. 1991. Peak heart rates during maximal running and swimming: implications for exercise prescription. *International Journal of Sports Medicine* 12: 309–12.

Fox III S.M., Naughton J.P., and Haskell, W.L. 1971. Physical activity and the prevention of coronary heart disease. *Annals of Clinical Research* 3:404–32.

Gibbons E.S. 1987. The significance of anaerobic threshold in exercise prescription. *Journal of Sports Medicine* 27: 357–61.

Goldberg L. et al. 1988. Assessment of exercise intensity formulas by use of ventilatory threshold. *Chest* 94 (1): 95–98.

Jones N.L. et al. 1982. *Clinical Exercise Testing.* 2nd edition. Philadelphia: W.B. Saunders & Co.

McGehee J., Tanner C., and Houmard J. 2005. A comparison of methods for estimating the lactate threshold. *The Journal of Strength and Conditioning Research* 19 (3): 553–58.

Mittleman M.A. et al. 1993. Triggering of acute myocardial infarction by heavy physical exertion. *New England Journal of Medicine* 329: 922.

Nicholls J.F., Phares S.L., and Buono M.J. 1997. Relationship between blood lactate response to exercise and endurance performance in competitive female master cyclists. *International Journal of Sports Medicine* 18: 458–63.

Pilegaard H., Juel C., and Wibrand E. 1993. Lactate transport studied in sarcolemmal giant vesicles from rats: effect of training. *American Journal of Physiology* 264: E156–60.

Robergs R.A. and Landwehr R. 2002. The surprising history of the "HRmax=220-age" equation. *Journal of Exercise Physiology* 5 (2): 1–10.

Sheffield L.T. et al. 1978. Maximal heart rate and treadmill performance of healthy women in relation to age. *Circulation* 57: 79–84.

Sjodin B., Jacobs I., and Svedenhag J. 1982. Changes in onset of blood lactate accumulation (OBLA) and muscle enzymes after training at OBLA. *European Journal of Applied Physiology* 49: 45–57.

Sue D.Y. et al. 1984. Normal values in adults during exercise testing. *Clinics in Chest Medicine* 5: 89–98.

Tanaka H., Monahan K.D., and Seals D.R. 2001. Age-predicted maximal heart rate revisited. *Journal of the American College of Cardiology* 37 (1): 153–56.

Vachon J.A., Bassett Jr D.R., and Clarke S. 1999. Validity of the heart rate deflection point as a predictor of lactate threshold during running. *Journal of Applied Physiology* 87 (1): 452–59.

Withers R.T., Sherman W.M., Miller J.M. and Costill D.L. 1981. Specificity of the anaerobic threshold in endurance-trained cyclists and runners. *European Journal of Applied Physiology* 47 (1): 93–104.

Wyatt F.B., Jackson C.G. and Tran Z.V. 1997. Metabolic threshold defined by disproportionate increases in physiological parameters: A meta-analytic review. *Medicine and Science in Sports and Exercise* 29 (5): S1342.

Zavorsky G.S. 2000. Evidence and possible mechanisms of altered maximum heart rate with endurance training and tapering. *Sports Medicine* 29 (1): 13–26.

CHAPTER 4

Anderson O. 2004. The search for the perfect intensity distribution. *Cycling Research News* 10 (2): 13–14.

Barbeau P., Serresse O., and Boulay M.R. 1993. Using maximal and submaximal aerobic variables to monitor elite cyclists during a season. *Medicine and Science in Sports and Exercise.* 25 (9): 1062–69.

Esteve-Lanao J., San Juan A.F., Earnest C.P., Foster

C., and Lucia A. 2005. How do endurance runners actually train? Relationship with competition performance. *Medicine and Science in Sports and Exercise* 37 (3): 496–504.

Jansson E. et al. 1978. Changes in muscle fiber type distribution in man after physical training. *Acta Physiologica Scandinavica* 104: 235.

Keren G. and Epstein Y. 1981. The effect of pure aerobic training on aerobic and anaerobic capacity. *British Journal of Sports Medicine* 15 (1): 27–29.

McLellan T.M. and Skinner J.S. 1982. Blood lactate removal during active recovery related to aerobic threshold. *International Journal of Sports Medicine* 3: 224.

O'Toole M.L., Douglas P.S., and Hiller W.D. Use of heart rate monitors by endurance athletes: lessons from triathletes. *Journal of Sports Medicine and Physical Fitness* 38 (3): 181–87.

Seiler K.S. and Kjerland G.O. 2004. Quantifying training intensity distribution in elite endurance athletes: is there evidence of an optimal distribution? *Scandinavian Journal of Medicine & Science in Sports*. In press.

Skinner J. and McLellan T. 1980. The transition from aerobic to anaerobic threshold metabolism. *Research Quarterly for Exercise & Sport* Sport 51: 234–48.

CHAPTER 5

Billat V.L., Demarle A., Slawinski J., Paiva M., and Koralsztein J.P. 2001. Physical and training characteristics of top-class marathon runners. *Medicine and Science in Sports and Exercise* 33 (12): 2089–97

Billat V.L., Flechet B., Petit B., Muriaux G., and Koralsztein J.P. 1999. Interval training at VO_2 max: Effects on aerobic performance and overtraining markers. *Medicine and Science in Sports and Exercise* 31 (1): 156–63.

Gaiga M.C. and Doherty D. 1995. The effect of an aerobic interval training program on intermittent anaerobic performance. *Canadian Journal of Applied Physiology* 20 (4): 452–64.

Hoffman P., Pokan R., Von Duvillard S.P., et al. 1997. Heart rate performance curve during incremental cycle ergometer exercise in healthy young male subjects. *Medicine and Science in Sports and*

Exercise 29: 762–68.

Lindsay F.H., Hawley J.A., Myburgh K.H., et al. 1996. Improved athletic performance in highly trained cyclists after interval training. *Medicine and Science in Sports and Exercise* 28 (11): 1427–34.

Robergs R.A. et al. 1991. Effects of warm-up on muscle glycogenolysis during intense exercise. *Medicine and Science in Sports and Exercise* 23: 7.

Safran M.R., Garrett Jr. W.E., Seaber A.V., et al. 1988. The role of warmup in muscular injury prevention. *The American Journal of Sports Medicine* 16 (20): 123–29.

Schumacher Y.O. and Mueller P. 2002. The 4000-m team pursuit cycling world record: theoretical and practical aspects. *Medicine and Science in Sports and Exercise* 34 (6): 1029–36.

Slawinski J., Demarle A., Koralsztein J.P., and Billat V. 2001. Effect of supra-lactate threshold training on the relationship between mechanical stride descriptors and aerobic energy cost in trained runners. *Archives of Physiology and Biochemistry* 109 (2): 110–16.

Weston A.R., Myburgh K.H., Lindsay F.H., et al. 1997. Skeletal muscle buffering capacity and endurance performance after high-intensity interval training by well- trained cyclists. *European Journal of Applied Physiology* 75 (1): 7–13.

CHAPTER 6

Bompa T.O. 1983. *Theory and Methodology of Training.* Kendall/Hunt Publishing: Dubuque, IA.

Bompa T.O. 1999. *Periodization: Theory and Methodology of Training.* Human Kinetics: Champaign, IL.

CHAPTER 7

Banister E.W., Calvert T.W., and Savage M.V. 1975. A systems model of training for athletic performance. *Journal of Sports Medicine* 7: 57–61.

Banister E.W. and Calvert T.W. 1980. Planning for future performance: implications for long term training. *Canadian Journal of Applied Physiology* 5 (3): 170–76.

Costill D.L., Flynn M.G., Kirwan J.P., Houmard J.A., Mitchell J.B., Thomas R., and Park S.H. 1988. Effects of repeated days of intensified training on muscle glycogen and swimming performance.

Medicine and Science in Sports and Exercise 20: 249–54.

Dimsdale J.E. et al. 1987. Postexercise peril: plasma catecholamines and exercise. *Journal of the American Medical Association* 251: 630.

Foster C., Hoyos J., Earnest C., and Lucia A. 2005. Regulation of energy expenditure during prolonged athletic competition. *Medicine and Science in Sports and Exercise* 37 (4): 670–75.

Fry R,W. 1991. Overtraining in athletes: An update. *Sports Medicine* 12: 32–65.

Hedelin R., Wiklund U., Bjerle P., and Henriksson-Larsen K. 2000. Short-term overtraining: effects on performance, circulatory responses, and heart rate variability. *Medicine and Science in Sports and Exercise* 32: 1480–84.

Hooper S.L. et al. 1995. Markers for monitoring overtraining and recovery. *Medicine and Science in Sports and Exercise* 27: 106.

Jeukendrup A.E., Hesselink M.K.C., Kuipers H., and Keizer H.A. 1992. Physiological changes in male competitive cyclists after two weeks of intensified training. *International Journal of Sports Medicine* 13: 534–41.

Koutedakis Y., Budgett R., and Faulmann L. 1990. Rest in underperforming elite competitors. *British Journal of Sports Medicine* 24 (4): 248–52.

Lehman M., Wieland H., and Gastmann U. 1997. Influence of an unaccustomed increase in training volume vs. intensity on performance, chematological and blood-chemical parameters in distance runners. *Journal of Sports Medicine and Physical Fitness* 37 (2): 110–16.

Morton R.H., Fitz-Clarke J.R., and Banister E.W. 1990. Modeling human performance in running. *Journal of Applied Physiology* 69 (3): 1171–77.

Nilson K., Schoene R.B., Robertson H.T., et al. 1981. The effect of iron repletion on exercise-induced lactate production in minimally iron deficient subjects. *Medicine and Science in Sports and Exercise* 13: 92.

O'Toole M.L., Douglas P.S., and Hiller W.D. 1998. Use of heart rate monitors by endurance athletes: lessons learned from triathletes. *Journal of Sports Medicine and Physical Fitness* 38 (3): 181–87.

Padilla S., Mujika I., Orbananos J., and Angulo F.

Exercise intensity during competition time trials in professional road cycling. *Medicine and Science in Sports and Exercise* 32 (4): 850–86.

Padilla S., Mujika I., Orbananos J., Santisteban J., Angulo F., and Jose Goiriena J. 2001. Exercise intensity and load during mass-start stage races in professional road cycling. *Medicine and Science in Sports and Exercise* 33 (5): 796–802.

Pichot V., Roche F., Gaspoz J.M., et al. 2000. Relation between heart rate variability and training load in middle-distance runners. *Medicine and Science in Sports and Exercise* 32 (10): 1729–36.

Snyder A.C., Jeukendrup A.E., Hesselink M.K., et al. 1993. A physiological/psychological indicator of over-reaching during intensive training. *International Journal of Sports Medicine* 14 (1): 29–32.

Stray-Gundersen J., Videman T., and Snell P.G. 1986. Changes in selected parameters during overtraining. *Medicine and Science in Sports and Exercise* 18: S54–55.

Urhausen A., Gabriel H.H., Weiler B., and Kindermann W. 1998. Ergometric and psychological findings during overtraining: a long-term follow-up study in endurance athletes. *International Journal of Sports Medicine* 19: 114–20.

Uusitalo A., Tahvanainen K., Uusitalo A., and Rusko H. 1996. Noninvasive evaluation of sympathovagal balance in athletes by time and frequency domain analyses of heart and blood pressure variability. *Clinical Physiology* 16: 575–88.

Volek, J. 1997. Influence of nutrition on anabolic hormone concentrations. *Strength & Health Report* 1 (7): 5.

Weltman A., Weltman J.Y., Schurrer R., et al. 1992. Endurance training amplifies the pulsatile release of growth hormone: effects of training intensity. *Journal of Applied Physiology* 72 (6): 2188–96.

Weltman A., Weltman J.Y., Womack C.J., et al. 1997. Exercise training decreases the growth hormone (GH) response to acute constant-load exercise. *Medicine and Science in Sports and Exercise* 29 (5): 669–76.

CHAPTER 8

Banister E.W., Carter J.B., and Zarkadas P.C. 1999.

Training theory and taper: validation in triathlon athletes. *European Journal of Applied Physiology* 79 (2): 182–91.

Beneke R. and Hutler M. 2005. The effects of training on running economy and performance in recreational athletes. *Medicine and Science in Sports and Exercise* 37 (10): 1794–99.

Brisswalter J., Legros P., and Durand M. 1996. Running economy, preferred step length correlated to body dimensions in elite middle distance runners. *Journal of Sports Medicine and Physical Fitness* 36: 7–15.

Costill D.L., King D.S., Thomas R., and Hargreaves M. 1985. Effects of reduced training on muscular power in swimmers. *Physiology and Sports Medicine* 13 (2): 94–101.

Fitts R.H., Costill D.L., and Gardetto P.R. 1989. Effect of swim-exercise training on human muscle fiber function. *Journal of Applied Physiology* 66: 465–75.

Fry R.W. 1992. Periodization and the presentation of overtraining. *Canadian Journal of Sports Science* 17: 241–48.

Fry R.W., Morton A.R., and Keast D. 1992. Periodization of training stress—a review. *Canadian Journal of Sports Science* 17: 234–40.

Gomes P.S. and Bhambhani Y. 1996. Time course changes and dissociation in VO_2 max at maximum and submaximum exercise levels as a result of training in males. *Medicine and Science in Sports and Exercise* 28 (5): 581.

Hickson R.C., Foster C., Pollock M.L., Galassi T.M., and Rich S. 1985. Reduced training intensities and loss of aerobic power, endurance, and cardiac growth. *Journal of Applied Physiology* 58: 492–99.

Hickson R.C. and Rosenkoetter M.A. 1981. Reduced training frequencies and maintenance of increased aerobic power. *Medicine and Science in Sports and Exercise* 13: 13–16.

Houmard J.A., Costill D.L., Mitchell J.B., Park S.H., Fink W.J., and Burns J.M. 1990. Testosterone, cortisol, and creatine kinase levels in male distance runners during reduced training. *International Journal of Sports Medicine* 11: 41–45.

Houmard J.A. 1991. Impact of reduced training on performance in endurance athletes. *Sports Medicine* 12 (6): 380–93.

Houmard J.A., Costill D.L., Mitchell J.B., Park S.H., Hickner R.C., and Roemmish J.N. 1990. Reduced training maintains performance in distance runners. *International Journal of Sports Medicine* 11: 46–51.

Houmard J.A. and Johns R.A. 1994. Effects of taper on swim performance. Practical implications. *Sports Medicine* 17 (4): 224–32.

Lehman M.J., Lormes W., Opitz-Gross A., et al. 1997. Training and overtraining: an overview and experimental results in endurance sports. *Journal of Sports Medicine and Physical Fitness* 37 (1): 7–17.

Neary J.P., Martin T.P., and Quinney H.A. 2003. Effects of taper on endurance cycling capacity and single muscle fiber properties. *Medicine and Science in Sports and Exercise* 35 (11): 1875–81.

Neary J.P., Martin T.P., Reid D.C., et al. 1992. The effects of a reduced exercise duration taper program on performance and muscle enzymes of endurance cyclists. *European Journal of Applied Physiology* 65: (1): 30–36.

Shepley B., MacDougall J.D., Cipriano N., et al. 1992. Physiological effects of tapering in highly trained athletes. *Journal of Applied Physiology* 72: 706–11.

Steinacker J.M., Lormes W., Lehmann M., and Altenburg D. 1998. Training of rowers before world championships. *Medicine and Science in Sports and Exercise* 30 (7): 1158–63.

Zarkadas P.C., Carter J.B., and Banister E.W. 1995. Modelling the effect of taper on performance, maximal oxygen uptake, and anaerobic threshold in endurance triathletes. *Advances in Experimental Medicine and Biology* 393: 179–86.

INDEX